YOUR BRAIN

ELECTRIC

Better Living through Neurochemistry

JAMES LEE

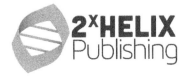

2×HELIX Publishing

This title was originally published as *Your Brain Electric.*
The title of the eBook version is –

Better Living through Neurochemistry

A guide to the optimization of serotonin, dopamine and the neurotransmitters that color your world

For information contact :
james@authorjameslee.com

ISBN-13: 978-1503072213
ISBN-10: 1503072215

CONTENTS

<u>Important Disclaimer</u>

The information provided in this book is designed to provide helpful information on the subjects discussed. This book is not meant to be used, nor should it be used, to diagnose or treat any medical condition. For diagnosis or treatment of any medical problem, consult your own veterinarian. The publisher and author are not responsible for any specific health or allergy needs that may require medical supervision and are not liable for any damages or negative consequences from any treatment, action, application or preparation, to any person reading or following the information in this book. References are provided for informational purposes only and do not constitute endorsement of any websites or other sources.

Preface

Notes Post-Publication

In the short period since the publication of this book, it has quickly gone on to becoming my second most popular book (behind *The Methuselah Project*). Typically, each book I write takes some time to gain traction and build word of mouth, however this book appeared to strike a chord from the day it was released.

As promised, I continue to stay abreast of the latest research into brain and body health. There are a few things I am investigating which will be included into this book in due course once I have been able to obtain further confirmation or additional analysis of clinical trial data.

However the single biggest update I have is regarding one of the most hated (and, it should be said, loved) drugs on the face of the planet – nicotine. Now, before you take your e-reader and hurl it across the room in disgust, hear me out. As someone who has witnessed the horror (and death too, unfortunately) of tobacco smoking, I was surprised to read some emerging research on nicotine. Recently, an expert whose opinion I value greatly said something that caught my ear. He mentioned that nicotine itself is actually an interesting and relatively benign drug – it's the delivery method (cigarettes) that "sucks" (his words). So, as someone with an unashamedly biased view against nicotine, I set about attempting to discern fact from fiction – and what I found was genuinely surprising. Nicotine (like most drugs, including caffeine, for example) is far from being completely harmless, with addiction risk remaining a factor even if it is determined to be beneficial for the brain. However it may surprise you to note that even nicotine's addictive qualities are being questioned, with many researchers now believing that much of tobacco's addictiveness comes from other substances found in the plant.

As nicotine's primary benefits are cognitive in nature (with the most noticeable effects being on concentration levels), I have covered this topic at greater length in my book *Brain Hacks*. However nicotine also appears to be a moderately potent way to boost dopamine. As I mention regularly, anything which boosts dopamine naturally creates an addictive quality, as dopamine is the neurochemical of reward and reinforcement. Whatever addictive qualities nicotine possesses will most likely occur through this pathway.

I cover this in the section on dopamine.

I want to stress that nothing in this book should constitute specific advice. It would be foolhardy for anyone to take advice from an eBook, just as it would be equally foolhardy for any author to think that they can give "one size fits all" advice to their readers. This is particularly the case for drugs with potential addiction risks including nicotine or ADHD drugs such as methylphenidate or dextroamphetamine. Any decision you or your doctor makes needs to be a *net* benefit for you. For example, for someone experiencing severe mood problems such as depression or anxiety, any risks or potential drug side-effects may seem small in comparison to the upside. On the other hand, the idea of taking powerful or addictive drugs to give yourself a little boost (or any other subtle desired effects) would seem ill-advised.

Introduction

For those fussy readers who "want to know what this book is about"[1]

There is a saying in science circles which says that if someone tells you they understand quantum physics, they *don't* understand quantum physics! Similarly, if someone tells you that "serotonin is the feel-good hormone" or "dopamine is the chemical of pleasure", they *don't* understand neurochemistry. Well, maybe it is part of the story but not the whole story as both of these neurotransmitters, along with many others, are responsible for a wide range of effects throughout your brain and

---

[1] I know, entitlement problem or what? I blame video games.

body.

Actually, the quantum physicals analogy is appropriate, as much of what happens inside your head operates more closely to the principles of quantum mechanics than it does to basic Newtonian physics. Rather than "if we do X then Y will occur", we have to talk the language of "action potentials", where particular chemical and electrical reactions occur without any fixed rule.

There are several reasons why I wrote this book. First and foremost, I have found that many people are interested in their own neurochemistry but are often scared off reading further by dense and boring textbooks on the topic. If you are ever having trouble sleeping, type in "serotonergic" into PubMed (where research trials and clinical reviews are published) and start reading. You will be asleep in minutes. So I want this book to serve as a tool to make what can often be a fascinating topic more accessible and entertaining.

Secondly, a sound understanding of basic neurochemistry and neurotransmission can quite often serve as an extremely useful diagnostic tool for your own particular mood or cognitive issues. Depression is an extremely common disorder, with around 5-10% of westerners clinically depressed at any one time and an amazing one out of four American women over the age of 50 currently on antidepressants.

When the average person visits their doctor suffering depression, they will invariably leave with a script for a drug which increases serotonin in the brain. This is despite the fact that there are a range of different neurochemical issues which can cause depression (or at least are associated with depression) and only some of which involve serotonin directly. The good news is that depression caused by low serotonin and depression caused by low dopamine or noradrenaline is usually strikingly different and fairly easy to identify if you know what you are looking for. So in this book I will give you all the information you need to know so you can easily tell the difference.

However I should also make another important point – *You are more than your neurotransmitters*. There is often a tendency to oversimplify what happens inside your head and to explain everything in terms of serotonin or dopamine. This is largely a construct of pharmaceutical companies whose self-serving "chemical imbalance" theory of anxiety and depression has become the default explanation when something goes awry inside our heads. There is no single illness called "depression" or "anxiety" and there are countless variations of each (as I will explain later). For example, whilst many people have depression caused by a lack of serotonin (or impaired serotonergic functioning), many do not. Depression can be caused by faulty thinking, life stressors, low dopamine, low noradrenaline, too much glutamate, thyroid problems and sleep disorders, to name but a few.

Considering this complexity, it is no surprise that there is no single treatment for all kinds of depression and anxiety. You have probably hear of SSRI drugs (*selective serotonin reuptake inhibitors* such as *Prozac*) which work by inhibiting the process by which your brain removes serotonin from the synapse (Don't worry, I will explain what synapses are also) and therefore keeping levels higher than they would have been. Sounds simple right? Well, did you know that there is another antidepressant drug called *Stablon* (tianeptine) which is a selective serotonin reuptake *enhancer*? Yes, that's right. Stablon does the exact opposite thing in your brain yet it also treats depression for some people.

First up I will give you a quick and dirty introduction to neurotransmission (Don't worry, I promise I won't bore you!) and then I will go into more detail on some of the main neurotransmitters in the brain which are relevant for mood disorders such as anxiety and depression.

Oh, and one more thing. As I have written a range of books and guides on various topics directly related to brain health and brain optimisation, whenever I mention a topic covered in greater detail in one of my other books, I will hyperlink it so you can click on the link and check it out to see if it interests you. Remember each book you purchase helps me make the repayments on my Maserati (Well, it's an 8 year old Mitsubishi, but I guess if you squint really hard it might look kinda Italian).

Let's begin, shall we?

Neuroscience 101

A boredom-free crash course to help you get the most out of this book

What is "neurotransmission"?

Neurotransmission is the mechanism your brain uses to send messages and trigger reactions by a kind of electrical transmission. Imagine a long line of people that stretches for miles. If someone at one end of the line wanted to get a message to the person at the other end, they would have one choice – *Chinese whispers*! That is how your brain communicates except that instead of people, you have individual neurons (brain cells) and instead of a whisper, each neuron releases a certain type of neurotransmitter to get the message across to the other neuron.

There is a gap between each neuron which is known as a *synapse* (or the *synaptic cleft*) and neurotransmitters are your brain's way of getting the message across the gap. The neurotransmitters are stored in vesicles (think of vesicles like little pouches) on the pre-synaptic neuron (the neuron sending the message is known as the *pre-synaptic neuron* and the neuron receiving the message is, unsurprisingly, known as the *post-synaptic neuron*).

Think of your neurotransmitters as keys which then need to open the right locks on the post-synaptic neuron. These locks are known as receptors. When a neurotransmitter binds to the receptor it triggers a reaction which then can often cascade through your nervous system using a kind of Chinese whispers system I mentioned earlier.

If you imagine a chain of neurons for a moment, it is easy to provide a simplified visualisation. Imagine the first neuron in the chain. It sends out a message using, say, serotonin, by sending it out via an axon (imagine a squid with tentacles – the axon is a tentacle that sends messages to nearby neurons). The serotonin will then bind to a specific receptor (called the *5-ht receptor*) on a tentacle on the receiving neuron called a dendrite. Axons send the message and dendrites receive.

There are a multitude of neurotransmitters and they are

generally classified as either excitatory or inhibitory. This doesn't necessarily mean that they make you "excited" (although neurotransmitters such as norepinephrine and dopamine certainly can), but means that they increase the chance that the neuron will then go on to fire an *action potential*. I would be at risk of boring you if I spent too much time getting into the detail of action potential, however suffice to say that when a neurotransmitter binds to a receptor, it is no guarantee of a predictable reaction, but a "potential" reaction. The key is for the neurochemical messenger received by the neuron to surpass a particular threshold of electrical activity. If it does so, an action potential will be triggered and if not, it won't.

The main excitatory neurotransmitters are glutamate, acetylcholine and norepinephrine (and epinephrine), while the primary inhibitory neurotransmitters are GABA and serotonin. Serotonin is actually a complicated one and is more accurately called a neuromodulator because, depending on the context, can be either excitatory or inhibitory. Despite this, by far the most common neurotransmitters in your nervous system are glutamate and GABA.

Modulating Neurotransmitter Activity with Drugs and Natural Substances

If you are reading this book, I am fairly confident that you have more than just a passing interest in fixing your own neurotransmitter activity or at least, optimising it. This can be a complicated topic so I have taken great pains to simplify this topic in the clearest possible terms. I also endeavour to be refreshingly clear of bias or a "fundamentalist" position. This is not a book where you will be told about the "evils" of "big pharma" or the apparently "magical" properties of various herbs and concoctions. Similarly, I will not try to tell you that all natural medicine is useless and that drugs are the only answer. You don't have to pick one or the other. You have the option of getting the best of both worlds.

However, I will be clear on one fairly reliable law of neurochemistry – If you are suffering from a severe issue (such as severe depression or anxiety), you will almost certainly require some kind of pharmacological assistance (along with everything else you will need to do to heal). For severe mental illness, supplements and herbal medicines don't cut it and those people recommending you stop your medication and go on a natural medicine are being reckless with other peoples' health. Likewise, for mild issues (mild anxiety, feeling sub-par and the like), antidepressants don't perform any better than a placebo. If you are in this scenario, it is likely that troubling side-effects would outweigh any benefits and you would be more likely to see results with particular natural therapies, along with the single greatest healer of neurochemical problems – exercise! (More on this later...)

Now, if, for some reason, you would like to increase levels of neurotransmitters such as serotonin, dopamine or noradrenaline, there are a limited number of pathways you can use to achieve this. This also leads to one of my bugbears with some proponents of natural therapies, who can sometimes make it seem like herbal medicines treat depression via some unique and separate pathway than that used by drugs. Popular herbal antidepressants such as St. John's Wort and Rhodiola Rosea treat depression the same way that certain drugs do, so the "natural" tag is, in some ways, a misnomer.

So, what are these ways we can increase levels of neurotransmitters? Let's use serotonin as an example to explain the various ways we can boost levels –

Inhibit the "re-uptake" process

When serotonin has done its job and triggered an action potential, your brain has a system for recycling it. There is a molecule known as the SERT (serotonin transporter) which acts like a bus that picks up the serotonin and takes it back to its "home base" neuron for processing. By blocking the action of SERT, more serotonin can build up in the synapse and hopefully, lead to improved mood or reduced anxiety.

This is how the popular SSRIs (selective serotonin re-uptake inhibitors such as Prozac and Zoloft) work. The main advantage of SSRIs over older antidepressants is that SSRIs are more "selective" (which should come as no surprise considering the name...) and therefore cause less side-effects. Some of the older antidepressants are subject to side-effects which can range from mildly troubling to life-threatening. However SSRIs are not without their own troubling side-effects, which include a constellation of problems from sexual dysfunction to diarrhoea.

The older class of antidepressants known as tricyclics also work in this way. This class, which includes drugs such as amitriptyline and clomipramine, is notorious for being un-selective (hence SSRIs are known as selective because they essentially target serotonin only) and therefore comes with a range of side-effects such as drowsiness. However their non-selectivity means that they are useful for a range of other applications such as amitriptyline's use for treating neuropathic pain and insomnia.

Block the action of the enzyme that breaks down serotonin

Another way serotonin is recycled after it has done its job is via an enzyme known as monoamine oxidase (MAO), which breaks down serotonin (as well as dopamine and noradrenaline) via an enzymatic process. Similarly to SSRIs, if you block this process, the serotonin doesn't get broken down at the same rate and then has a chance to build up in the synapse.

Drugs that do this are called MAOIs (monoamine oxidase inhibitors) and were an older class of medications that are rarely used these days due to safety concerns. The main problem with MAOIs is that they require dietary restrictions. If someone taking a MAOI consumes food or drink high in tyramine (such as aged cheese), it can trigger a massive spike in blood pressure and can lead to death. So it's not surprising that these have been largely ditched since the advent of SSRIs, which are virtually impossible to overdose on or accidentally kill yourself with.

That said, many experts believe that MAOIs remain the most effective antidepressant drugs to this day and they are therefore used occasionally with those who don't respond to other drugs. If you are in a deep dark hole the, according to certain experts, your best bet is either MAOIs or ECT (electroconvulsive therapy).

Stimulating the receptor

Substances known as receptor agonists can artificially activate receptors, triggering the effects that would occur if the neurotransmitter itself did the job. For certain receptor types, this is a simple proposition, whereas for others, things get a little complicated. For example, opiate drugs such as morphine and codeine function as opiate agonists, mimicking the action of natural endorphins and consequently reducing pain. The class of anti-anxiety (and sleep) medications known as benzodiazepines (such as Xanax, Temazepam and Valium) act as GABA receptor agonists and therefore calm you down.

However serotonin receptors are a little more complicated and this is the reason why there are no effective antidepressants which operate primarily as serotonin receptor agonists. This is because there are a range of sub-types of the serotonin receptor and each sub-type has different effects when activated. For example, activating the 5-HT_{1A} receptor can reduce anxiety (such as the drugs buspirone and trazodone), whereas activating 5-HT_{2A} (such as psychedelics such as LSD do) can make you believe that there is a clown in your closet who wants you dead. Or alternatively, activating 5-HT_{1B} (as the triptan class of drugs do) will treat migraines and cluster headaches. If you go messing around with serotonin, you'd better make sure you target the right receptor!

Then there are inverse agonists which agonise the receptor to trigger the exact opposite effect as a direct agonist would.

In case you were wondering, yes, serotonin and other neurotransmitters are classified as agonists of their relevant receptors.

Blocking the receptor

A receptor antagonist (or a receptor blocker) occupies the receptor and prevents the endogenous (natural/non-pharmacological) neurotransmitter from doing its job.

Of all the various ways you can modulate receptor activity, antagonism can be the most confusing to understand because of the different ways that different types of receptors (and neurotransmitters) respond to antagonism. For example, the common class of anti-hypertensive drugs (to reduce blood pressure) known as beta-blockers block the beta-adrenal receptors and reduce blood pressure (by reducing adrenal activation of those receptors. However, there are a class of antidepressants which act as serotonin receptor antagonists (such as mirtazapine). How can a drug which blocks serotonin treat depression? This is actually a very long story and I would run the real risk of boring you to death so I will give you the "digest" version. Firstly, there are many researchers who dispute whether serotonin receptor antagonists even increase serotonergic neurotransmission. This is backed up by the fact that antagonists such as mirtazapine don't cause any of the effects typically associated with increased serotonin (such as serotonin syndrome or sexual dysfunction). However other researchers believe that antagonists increase serotonin by blocking the sub-types which increase anxiety and depression and thereby increasing activity of the unaffected sub-types.

Stimulating neurotransmitter release[2]

The other way we can increase levels of serotonin and other neurotransmitters is to force the presynaptic neuron to release its stores. Imagine the serotonin is sitting in a bag hanging from the roof. This is the equivalent of squeezing on the bag to force the contents out.

In the case of serotonin, the most potent releasing agent is the drug ecstasy which basically drains your brain of not only serotonin but also tryptophan, the amino acid precursor. This is

---

[2] Or inhibiting its storage in the vesicle.

why, unsurprisingly, you feel rather depressed after an ecstasy "trip". As a side note, next time someone tries to tell you that depression has nothing to do with serotonin, you can helpfully point out ecstasy, where serotonin depletion causes a perfect analogue of depression (albeit for a few days only). (Note – As I will mention repeatedly, this does not mean that all depression is caused by serotonin. There is depression cause by low dopamine and a multitude of other causes. However depression related to low serotonin is undeniably common. I should also point out that we don't yet know whether low serotonin causes depression or is the result of depression. That's how complicated this picture is!)

The most common releasing agents are the amphetamine class of drugs and the ADHD medication methylphenidate (Ritalin). Amphetamines powerfully trigger the release of noradrenaline, dopamine and serotonin. Considering such powerful action on all three of your key mood related neurotransmitters (with the exception of opiate receptors perhaps), it is not hard to see why drugs like methamphetamine (meth) are so addictive.

In general, releasing agents are fraught with danger because they tend to rob future neurotransmitters to feed the present. For example, reuptake inhibitors gradually increase serotonin over time, whereas releasing agents dump everything into the synapse, leaving none for tomorrow. This means, as a general rule regarding depression and anxiety, releasing agents make you feel much better today and then much worse tomorrow as your brain just can't replenish levels of neurotransmitters quickly enough to keep up.

What about "natural" substances?

If you are considering a natural alternative to a particular drug, you need to bear in mind that, in general, most supplements and herbs will work in the same basic ways mentioned above. And when you read about a particular supplement being "milder" with less side-effects, sometimes it can mean that there are no positive effects either.

Essentially, natural antidepressants work as either mild SSRIs or mild MAOIs, with often conflicting research as to which. For example, researchers are currently divided as to whether St. John's Wort is an SSRI or a MAOI. At the end of the day, this is relatively unimportant. More pertinent is whether sometime works or not. The only exception to this is when you are suffering from low dopamine. SSRIs tend to suppress dopaminergic function whereas MAOIs give all three mood-related monoamine neurotransmitters a boost. So if low dopamine is an issue, you would either need to focus on a supplement that purely works on dopamine (such as mucuna pruriens) or a MAOI like rhodiola rosea.

Next, let's dive deeper into often treacherously ill-defined waters.

Why are clinical trials of antidepressant drugs and supplements so underwhelming?

Poor clinical trial results of both drugs and supplements used to treat mood disorders are often used by one side to tackle the other. Naturopaths point out that SSRIs only work for a small percentage of patients, while doctors do the same for supplements. In my view, this is simply further evidence of the fact that what we call "depression" or "generalized anxiety" is not one illness, but a cluster of symptoms that help us to at least get a rough idea of what is wrong. Just as there are myriad forms of depression, so are there myriad causes.

If a company were to develop a drug which cured (for example) multiple sclerosis (MS) by repairing myelin, if 100 people entered a trial, you would expect the vast majority (minus a small number of people whose bodies blocked the process by some rare quirk) to improve dramatically. However if you place 100 people with depression into a trial for a new SSRI, you would expect that the only ones to improve would be those whose depression is serotonergic in nature. It wouldn't help those whose depression is related to dopamine, noradrenaline, NMDARs, cortisol or any of the other common causes of depression.

So the best any drug or supplement can hope for is a small benefit which is statistically significant, meaning (in this context) that the result is unlikely to be caused by placebo effect. Hence why I recommend people make up their own mind by looking at statistical significance, not the overall proportion of people who benefit. I am also pragmatic regarding the power of anecdotes. So whilst you should never base your view solely on anecdotes, they have undeniable power. Anyone who writes non-fiction knows the power of the anecdote if you wish to engage the reader. People love a narrative. A single line of narrative can have more impact than reams of data. Whether or not scientists like to admit it, for someone who is depressed, their friend telling them that "Supplement X" or "Drug X" *"literally cured my depression"* is significantly more powerful than –

A total of 255 patients who met the DSM-IV major or minor depressive disorder and recently developed ACS were randomly assigned to the escitalopram (n=127) or placebo (n=128) group in this 24-week double-blind trial (ClinicalTrial.gov identifier: NCT00419471). Remission was defined as a Hamilton Rating Scale for Depression (HAMD) score ≤7. Assays were performed for the 5-HTTLPR, STin2 VNTR, 5-HTR2a 102T/C, and 5-HTR2a 1438A/G genotypes. Escitalopram was superior to placebo for treating depressive disorder with ACS but there were no significant associations between serotonergic genes and treatment responses even when considering ACS severity[3].

---

[3] Psychiatry Investig. 2016 Jan;13(1):157-60. doi: 10.4306/pi.2016.13.1.157.

Serotonin

Happy, calm and content

Serotonin is a monoamine neurotransmitter involved in a range of functions including mood, appetite, sleep, digestion. Serotonin is known as the "feel-good hormone", however the majority of all serotonin in your body is located in your gut, where it drives the process of digestion.

Impaired serotonergic function is associated with:

- Low mood
- Anxiety
- Sleeping problems (insomnia, poor quality sleep)
- Aggression
- Increased pain
- Digestive problems (constipation, diarrhoea, stomach

pains)

The good news is that issues related to low serotonin are relatively easy to fix with either drugs, supplements or cognitive and behavioral changes. However it is not all good news and there are a few things you should note.

Serotonin problems are slow to fix and just replenishing serotonin doesn't cure depression.

One of the great mysteries of pharmacology is why it takes up to 3 months to improve when someone takes an antidepressant like an SSRI, as serum levels of serotonin (measured via metabolites) only take around 3 days to normalise. This is due to several reasons.

When you restore serotonin levels via drug therapy, it triggers (perhaps indirectly) a gradual healing process that can take a long time. Firstly, we have the issue of receptor down-regulation and up-regulation. When there is low serotonergic activity for a long period of time, serotonin receptors up-regulate, which means, they become much better at utilising the limited supply of serotonin more efficiently. However, when you start taking an SSRI, it triggers an interesting process which many researchers believe is the reason why a small minority of people commit suicide shortly after starting an antidepressant.

The first thing that happens is that your brain, through special receptors, senses that there is ample serotonin available and throttles back production and release. This can then send someone into a temporary yet intensely unpleasant black hole as their brain then starts to adjust. Beginning an antidepressant is often a case of "two steps forward, one step back". It is fascinating that most people I have dealt with or followed on various discussion forums have followed an almost identical timeline:

- **Day 1-3** – Increased anxiety as the drug gives an almost stimulant effect.
- **Day 3-7** – Happier than they have been since becoming ill. Sometimes almost euphoric as their serotonin levels spike.
- **Week 2-3** – Mood drops again as the brain throttles serotonergic activity. This can either be a minor drop in mood or suicidally bad, depending on the person. If this is you, the key point to raise here is not to give up hope. I think many people just assume they are about to fall back into a black hole again and never come out. This kind of thinking could reasonably lead to suicidal thoughts.
- **Week 3-12** – Gradual improvement and by the third month will start to think of themselves as "back to normal".

However as you probably know, not everyone responds to antidepressants and this leads to the second complicating point with treating problems with serotonin. Firstly, as I have already mentioned, not all depression is caused by serotonergic issues. So someone with a kind of *anhedonic* (inability to feel pleasure) depression caused by low dopamine would not show the same recovery timeline as the example above. This is one of the problems with the modern obsession drug companies have with serotonin. For example, the only option at present for someone with depression caused by low dopamine is either an old-school MAOI or the smoking cessation aid bupropion (*Wellbutrin* when used for depression and *Zyban* when used for quitting smoking).

Secondly, even if serotonin is behind your depression (or anxiety), it is not simply a case of filling up the tank and away we go. There are countless ways your serotonin system can get out of whack. Some of the more common are:

- Not enough serotonin being released by the presynaptic neuron
- Your re-uptake process is too quick, leaving too little serotonin in the synapse
- Your MAO activity is too high, breaking down serotonin too quickly
- You are not consuming enough tryptophan in your diet, so your brain cannot produce enough serotonin
- You are consuming enough tryptophan however your body is inefficient at converting it into serotonin
- You are consuming a diet high in tyrosine relative to tryptophan. Tyrosine is the amino acid precursor to dopamine and noradrenaline and it competes with tryptophan to cross the blood brain barrier (the barrier which protects your brain from various alien substances).

And this is just looking at the biochemical pathways. Possibly more relevant is looking at the various cognitive and behavioral processes that send serotonin levels lower. A stressful life or a dead-end job will mess up serotonin more swiftly than any of the pathways mentioned above. More on this in a moment.

So naturally, depending on your particular quirks, different treatments will have different outcomes. For example, on many forums you will see people claiming that tryptophan or 5-htp (5-htp is another supplement which is one step closer to serotonin, biochemically) are effective antidepressants. If low levels of tryptophan are behind your particular issues, then this will be the case. However if you are depressed, yet have no issues with tryptophan, taking these types of supplements will be unlikely to help.

So this process can become one of trial and error as you experiment with what works and what doesn't work. As I have mentioned many times in my books, I am always about simplification and distilling everything down to key points, so I would like to summarise the process of fixing serotonergic issues like this:

- Fix the neurochemistry via drugs or supplements. If you are suffering from mild depression or anxiety, look towards supplements. If you are suffering from moderate to severe depression or anxiety, consider pharmacological options.
- Fix the behaviors that suppress or deplete serotonin
- Fix the faulty thinking that suppresses or depletes serotonin.

Drug-based options for boosting serotonin

By far the most common way people boost serotonin is via SSRI antidepressants, however there are other ways of achieving this in the event that SSRIs don't work for you or if they have side-effects which led you to cease use. This means we need to refer to the basics of neurochemistry mentioned earlier. There is more than one way to relieve a cat of its fur, and there are more ways to boost serotonin.

However it would be sensible to begin with the class of drugs a reader is most likely to use (or at least start with).

Selective serotonin re-uptake inhibitors (SSRIs)

SSRIs are popular for good reason. They are safe and relatively effective. They are therefore typically your doctor's first option when they suspect you have low serotonin. However I should point out that they are far from perfect. As mentioned earlier, they only work for some people and for others the side-effects can be unbearable (yet others experience either mild side-effects or none whatsoever). The most common side effects of SSRIs are –

- Sexual dysfunction (lack of libido, problems achieving an erection and inability to orgasm)
- Sleep disturbances (These tend to be more common at the start of therapy)
- Blunted mood – This means that you feel a bit flat or don't get excited about anything. As SSRIs tend to keep people

in a narrower mood band (thus preventing severe mood swing), this is not surprising.

It should also be pointed out that, for some people, coming off SSRIs (and other antidepressants also) can be hellish. If and when you need to stop SSRI therapy, you need to taper off the drug very, very slowly to minimise discontinuation syndrome.

Another thing to bear in mind is that, whilst all SSRIs work in roughly the same way, different people respond to different types, so sometimes some trial and error is required. You only have to type in (for example) "Lexapro user reviews" into Google to see this in action. For some, Lexapro changes their life and cures their depression, whereas for others it either does nothing or puts them through hell. Same goes for all of the SSRIs, so you can see how important it can often be to try a different one if the one you start with doesn't work. Just because you read someone on a forum claim that one particular SSRI is the "best", that doesn't mean the same will apply in your case.

The main SSRIs used today are –

- **Lexapro** (escitalopram)
- **Cipralex** (citalopram)[4]
- **Zoloft** (sertraline)
- **Paxil** (paroxetine)

---

[4] Note – Escitalopram is the updated version of citalopram, however it doesn't necessarily mean that in your case escitalopram will work better. However in general, these two are virtually identical in terms of effects, with escitalopram having a slightly better side-effect profile)

- **Prozac** (fluoxetine)

There is also another related class known as SNRIs (serotonin and noradrenaline re-uptake inhibitors) which act in the same manner as SSRIs, but also have effects on noradrenaline. The two main available SNRIs are –

- **Venlafaxine (Effexor)**
- **Desvenlafaxine** (Pristiq – A long half-life version of Effexor which enables you to only have to take one per day and it lasts until the next day)
- **Cymbalta** (duloxetine)

Again, whether you need an SSRI or an SNRI will largely come down to trial and error, however some doctors have found that, due to the extra effects on noradrenaline, SNRIs can be helpful where there is a lack of energy. On the other hand, in cases where there is already anxiety present, SNRIs can sometimes make the situation worse.

Tricyclics (TCAs)

The best way to think of these older class of antidepressants is like a "less specific SNRI". Whereas SNRIs can, fairly cleanly, target serotonin and noradrenaline only, tricyclics affect many other systems in the brain at the same time. This can be good and bad.

The main benefit of tricyclics' messy effects is that they can then be used to treat other conditions which respond to one of these effects. For example, amitriptyline blocks neuropathic pain signals so can be used to treat conditions such as fibromyalgia. Amitriptyline (along with several other tricyclics) also acts as a sedating antihistamine so can be used as a sleep aid.

Unfortunately it is not all good news. The greatest single difference between tricyclics and SSRIs is that, if you were insane enough to consume an entire packet (or jar) of SSRIs, you would probably live. If you did the same with tricyclics, you would probably die. In large doses, tricyclics are cardiotoxic, which, as you probably guessed, means they are not good for your heart in higher doses. They also come with a jaw-dropping long list of side-effects such as sedation and weight gain. These side-effects are not to be sniffed at and cause many people to stop taking them.

The other obvious problem is, because they increase serotonin and noradrenaline at the same time, if you want to just raise serotonin, most of them lack sufficient specificity to do this. That said, some of them (such as clomipramine) are significantly potent at increasing serotonin but less so for noradrenaline, so there are options within the class.

Tricyclics are serious drugs. They are not drugs to take if you are feeling "a little off" or looking for a "pick me up". They are potent drugs with a range of side-effects. However on the flipside, for some they can be lifesavers. Particularly those that haven't responded to SSRIs for whatever reason. For example, many experts believe that, despite the advent of SSRIs, tricyclics like clomipramine, imipramine and amitriptyline remain the most effective antidepressants available. You just have to pay the piper in terms of side-effects.

Serotonin-releasing agents

As mentioned earlier, serotonin releasing agents are, in general, not sustainable options for increasing levels of serotonin as they tend to dump serotonin into your synapses at the expense of tomorrow. This is why they are not typically used as antidepressants. Oh, and there is the small issue of the most potent serotonin releaser – MDMA (ecstasy) being illegal. There is considerable debate as to whether MDMA has a role to play in legal pharmacotherapy however. Proponents (including some psychotherapists) believe that MDMA can be helpful in certain therapeutic circumstances. Other researchers point out that, in (extremely) high doses, MDMA has been shown to be neurotoxic for mice – and there are more than a few ex-ravers out there who have fried their serotonin receptors after years of abusing this drug. The truth probably lies somewhere in the middle. In fact, in the UK a few years back, Professor David Nutt (who was the government's chief advisor on drugs and drug policy) was sacked for suggesting that MDMA was less harmful than alcohol!

The only legal serotonin releasing agent available (the pain reliever tramadol) is also fraught with danger as it also has a mild opiate agonist action, making it potentially addictive for some. I actually have a vaguely controversial opinion regarding tramadol. It is one of the few legally available drugs which you can take and it improves your mood within a few hours. As you know, antidepressants take weeks to lift your mood. This is because tramadol does a few things as the same time, making it quite an interesting drug. Among other things it acts as a –

- Serotonin releasing agent (improving mood)
- Noradrenaline re-uptake inhibitor (gives you energy and lifts mood)
- Opiate agonist (dulls both mental and physical pain)
- NMDA antagonist (NMDA antagonists are the latest subject of research into new antidepressants as certain NMDA antagonists such as ketamine have been shown to lift depression in hours, not weeks!)

I believe there is a role to play for a drug like tramadol, if respected appropriately and only in very specific circumstances. There is a growing band of people claiming that when nothing else worked, tramadol lifted them out of their dark hole. However I should also point out that there is an equally large group of people telling of the horrors of quitting either large doses or long term use. This is another drug not to be trifled with and I am still not convinced of its effectiveness as a long term treatment for depression, due to the serotonin releasing properties.

Serotonin receptor antagonists and agonists

The theory behind these drugs is quite seductive and would appear to suggest that this is a promising way to increase levels of serotonin. However, unfortunately, I, along with many researchers and clinicians remain unconvinced as to the ability of antagonists and agonists to increase levels of serotonin.

There are several pieces of key evidence that show us why this is the case. Firstly, this class of drug is relatively ineffective for treating severe depression, anxiety or obsessive compulsive disorder (OCD). This is particularly the case with OCD as there is a clear relationship between the potency of a particular drug at increasing levels of serotonin and its ability to treat OCD. For example, probably the best drug for OCD is clomipramine, which is also one of the most potent agents available for increasing serotonin. While antagonists and agonists can be useful additions to an SSRI for depression or anxiety (For example – mirtazapine is fantastic for improving sleep and reducing sexual dysfunction for those on an SSRI), they are rarely a doctor's first or central option for treating these conditions.

Secondly, this class of drug does not display any of the tell-tale signs typically associated with serotonergic drugs. This is a point often repeated by respected researcher Dr Ken Gillman, who points out that it is impossible to give yourself serotonin syndrome by taking large doses of mirtazapine, or combining mirtazapine with other serotonergic drugs. As Dr Gillman points out, increasing serotonin is associated with reliable symptoms such as sexual dysfunction, however mirtazapine has the exact *opposite* effect and can actually be a *treatment* for sexual dysfunction!

So in general, if you are looking at increasing levels of

serotonin, there are much better options. In the example of mirtazapine, the only exception I can think of is where low serotonin is being caused by sleep dysfunction or not eating properly. As mirtazapine is a wonderful sleep aid (mainly by increasing slow wave/deep sleep) and can make you eat like a horse, it could indirectly contribute to normalizing serotonin this way.

Natural and drug-free options for boosting serotonin

As I try to make clear throughout my books, I would characterize my position on drugs versus "natural" as *pragmatic*. I have always found it rather perplexing that most books on this topic are either one or the other, but rarely both. Or more specifically, these books *advocate* for one or the other, often giving dogmatic, "one size fits all" views to their readers. It is perfectly fine to focus on one or the other for the purposes of giving readers targeted information. My book Chill Pills and Mood Food was an example of this, focusing on natural ways to boost mood and reduce anxiety. The difference is that I avoid making your decision for you by telling you what you should and shouldn't use. Information is power, so I always follow the "teach a man to fish..." principle, rather than making peoples' decisions for them. Accordingly, I like to think that I provide balanced insight, relatively free of dogma.

When used correctly and in the right context, natural

serotonin boosters can be a fantastic option for gently increasing levels over time. However the problem is that often they are not used for the right reasons or in the right occasions. If you are severely depressed, forget about using supplements and herbs, as they are unlikely to provide sufficient relief. Severe depression (particularly with any suicidal ideation) is not something to mess around with. Almost always, severe depression will respond best to a combination of medication, CBT (cognitive behavioral therapy) and physical exercise. Then, if your doctor agrees, once you are able to come off the medication, you could consider a mild, natural option as a kind of "maintenance therapy" to keep serotonin levels up. On the flipside, medication is complete overkill for mild depression and anxiety. This is where natural options shine. If you are feeling a bit flat or out of sorts, natural options (along with physical exercise of course!) can be wonderful for getting you back in the game. Medications come with a range of side-effects that could make you even more depressed, whereas if you are severely depressed, these side-effects are a small price to pay for recovery.

At the risk of heading into broken record territory, there is no "best" when deciding on whether you want to go down the natural route, or whether you feel that your situation may require more urgent relief. There is only what's right for *you*.

This seems to me to be such common sense that I am always shocked to read fundamentalist views by both sides of the "Drug v Natural" debate. On one side you have homeopaths and some of the less scrupulous naturopaths telling severely depressed "patients" to stop taking their medication – often with disastrous effects. On the other side you have doctors who think that anything "natural" is all just hocus pocus. The truth lies, as it usually does in most cases, somewhere in the middle of this debate.

In terms of natural options, there are a few gold-standard supplements which are already widely used, along with one or two newer options which are beginning to gain recognition. I have mentioned this elsewhere previously, however it is important to point out that countless plants have biological actions which modulate neurotransmitters. So when you see it mentioned that *Plant X* or *Herb X* "increases serotonin", it is important to elucidate whether or not the increase in serotonin is significant. This is why St. John's Wort is so widely used; it has a startlingly potent effect on serotonin levels compared to most other non-pharmaceutical options (although still substantially less than even the weakest SSRI, used at typical dosages).

This being the case, there are only a handful of natural substances which have enough serotonergic effect to be considered relevant or useful. On top of those mentioned, there are one or two others which show promise, while needing more research. These include:

St. John's Wort (Hypericum)

St. John's Wort is the undisputed king of herbal antidepressants for good reason. It potently increases levels of serotonin, has a long history of widespread use (making clinical studies more statistically significant) and is associated with none of the severe side-effects usually associated with pharmacological antidepressants.

St. John's Wort (or *hypericum perforatum*) is a perennial flowering herb native to Europe and some parts of Asia and Africa. It is easily recognised due to its beautiful yellow flowers. Yes, the yellow flowers have nothing to do with how it works as an antidepressant however if you are an avid gardener in the right geography, I highly recommend trying to grow St. John's Wort - it looks amazing in my own garden!

St. John's Wort has an impressive body of individual research studies and meta-analyses (where groups of studies are pooled together for better statistical significance) backing its use for mild to moderate depression, including -

- A 1995 meta-analysis of twelve individual trials founds that hypericum was significantly superior to a placebo (an "inert" sugar pill with no active ingredients) and as effective as modern pharmaceuticals at relieving depression. (This study didn't say whether it was severe or mild depression)
- A 1996 meta-analysis found that hypericum was almost three times more effective than placebo, with an efficacy that matched tricyclic antidepressants for the treatment of

mild to moderate depression. Not only this, but hypericum was found to be significantly safer and with much milder side-effects.

- A more recent meta-analysis with stricter criteria was a little more subdued, albeit still with a positive outcome. This trial found that hypericum was 1.5 times as effective as placebo, but also concluded that hypericum was as effective as tricyclic drugs.

- Another study concluded that, while hypericum was effective for treating mild to moderate depression, it was slightly less effective than tricyclic drugs.

- A 1999 study found that hypericum was as effective as Prozac (fluoxetine) for the treatment of mild to moderate depression in the elderly.

The other major component of hypericum's mode of action is its ability to also concurrently treat the biomarkers of chronic stress. Stress and depression go hand in hand. It is often after a period of unrelenting stress that depression can result. Hypericum has been testing on rodents, where they are given hypericum before being subjected to various stressful situations (as an aside, everyone should take a moment to thank all these poor rodents that suffer so that we might not). In all the various measurements of stress response, hypericum has been shown to reduce the biomarkers of stress, such as cortisol levels.

Depression and chronic stress is also often associated with disturbances in the HPA (hypothalamus pituitary adrenal) axis, your brain's (and body's) system for dealing with stress. Hypericum has also been shown to positively modulate that HPA axis, leading to amelioration of certain aspects of acute and chronic stress.

It is important to note that a large number of people who start drug therapy soon quit due to intolerable side-effects. In many cases, these side-effects eventually settle down and fade, however for many people it is too hard to bear and they quit. Natural therapies such as hypericum have a much gentler start-up period, which means that, although it can take a little longer to have noticeable effects, people are unlikely to quit due to side-effects. I should also point out that this longer start-up period is another reason why natural options are not appropriate for more severe cases. If someone is severely depressed or even suicidal, their physician needs to choose the therapy that will pull them out of their deep, dark hole the most quickly. Unfortunately, I would never, ever recommend natural therapies in such acute cases. If this describes you, please put down this eBook and seek immediate, professional attention. There are powerful, effective treatments that can quickly treat your current condition.

Unfortunately there is no consensus as to exactly how hypericum exerts its beneficial effects on depression. Some researchers have claimed that it works as an SSRI, while others have indicated that it works as a MAOI. An *in-vitro* (i.e. - in a laboratory test-tube, not in an animal or human) study in 1994 found that hypericum clearly inhibited the action of monoamine oxidase when used at high doses. Similarly, studies conducted in 1997 and 1998 using even higher doses found that hypericum works at least partially as a MAOI. The problem with these high-dose studies is that they found no inhibition of monoamine oxidase using clinically relevant doses (i.e. - doses which roughly approximate what a person would typically take). So, while we know that hypericum functions as MAOI to at least some extent, it is unclear from these studies whether it functions as a MAOI at the dosages people are likely to take.

Likewise, several German studies in the 1990s found that hypericum inhibits the re-uptake of serotonin, norepinephrine and dopamine in-vitro, in a similar fashion to pharmaceutical antidepressants.

Animal studies have also all found a variety of effects, with no clear indication of a single mechanism underlying how exactly hypericum works. However the key point to draw from these and other studies is that hypericum consistently increases levels of serotonin, norepinephrine and dopamine in the brain. It's just that the relative degree to which each of these monoamines is increased or the proposed mechanism differs between studies. Of these, it appears as if serotonin is most affected, which is why I have included hypericum in this section.

While hypericum is generally an effective and potent natural antidepressant, it has one major downside - it affects how your body metabolises a variety of drugs. In fact, hypericum appears to affect almost any drug that is metabolised in the liver. Of particular concern is the impact on the blood-thinning drug warfarin. Depending on the drug, hypericum can either increase or decrease the effectiveness of the particular medication. Therefore, if you are on any drugs at all, you need to clear things with your doctor before taking hypericum. In general however, I usually recommend that, if someone is taking any other medication, to first investigate curcumin and/or rhodiola rosea, as these don't have the same effects on other drugs

The only other potential side effect of note is increased photosensitivity. In a practical sense, this means that some people can become sunburned much more quickly than otherwise would have been the case if they were not taking hypericum. So I think it would be warranted to take a little extra precaution regarding sun exposure if you are taking hypericum.

Also, I should point out that you should never combine hypericum with pharmaceutical antidepressants or any other drug that increases levels of serotonin, norepinephrine or dopamine. This can, in rare cases, lead to a life-threatening condition called serotonin syndrome. If in doubt, discuss with your primary care physician.

Rhodiola rosea

Rhodiola is a supplement I have been passionate about for a long time now, due to its unique mechanism of action and wide-ranging effects. Along with curcumin, rhodiola is one of my picks for supplements which will become increasingly well-known over the next ten years or so.

As with hypericum and curcumin, I have chosen to include rhodiola in the section on serotonin as that is where there appears to be the most potent effects. However each of these also increases dopamine, so in mild cases where both dopamine and serotonin are lowered, these three supplements can all be great options.

Rhodiola rosea is an herbal supplement which has been used for decades in Russian-block countries to treat what they refer to as *'nervous disorders'*, which encapsulates a range of conditions including stress, anxiety and depression. However it has only recently risen to prominence in the West. Rhodiola rosea (also known as *golden root* or *arctic root*, among other things) is a plant that grows in cold areas of the northern hemisphere and is most commonly associated with countries such as Russia and the other countries of the former USSR and has been reputedly used extensively by the Russian military to promote endurance.

In terms of prominence in the west, rhodiola rosea still lags far behind St. John's Wort, which enjoys far more popularity and widespread use. This is a pity, because rhodiola has a few advantages over St. John's Wort (which I will get to in a moment).

Rhodiola rosea belongs to a class of herbs known as *adaptogens*. Adaptogens are substances which restore homeostasis in the body. So if, for example, you are too wired and anxious, an adaptogen will calm you down. If you are lethargic and lacking energy, an adaptogen will give you energy.

Quite often, I am rather suspicious of adaptogens and the theory that underpins this class of supplements. There are quite a few natural therapies marketed as adaptogens which have very poor research-based evidence backing their use. However rhodiola is one herbal medicine where there is not only a large body of anecdotal reports verifying the adaptogenic effects, but a good theoretical potential mechanism that would explain the effects.

By increasing levels of serotonin, norepinephrine and dopamine, rhodiola functions in a very similar way to a pharmaceutical antidepressant. If you are *anxious depressed* (high stress, high anxiety, poor sleep) and you take an antidepressant (such as an SSRI, tricyclic or MAOI) you will usually slowly begin to calm down and relax over time. If you are suffering from a more lethargic depression (low energy, hypersomnia, lack of motivation) and you take the same antidepressant, you will gradually start to spark up and feel more energetic. It is for this reason that, when people talk of the adaptogenic properties of rhodiola, what I believe they are really referring to is its ability to act as an antidepressant by increasing levels of the three primary monoamines.

Due to the fact that rhodiola increases levels of all three monoamines (as it acts as a MAOI), it tends to be a little more "activating" than St. John's Wort. Not surprisingly, I have therefore found it more helpful in cases of lethargic depression, rather than anxious depression.

The beauty of several antidepressant supplements such as rhodiola and curcumin, is that they function as MAOIs but without the dangerous dietary risks. This is important to note, because without the danger component, MAOIs are excellent for treating depression due to their broad range of action.

Due to the comparative lack of drug interactions, I usually recommend rhodiola rosea as the first option for treating depression if someone decides to go down the natural route. As it is a slightly newer supplement in the west, there isn't as much research yet compared to St. John's Wort, however what research is available has been generally positive. In particular, multiple rodent trials have demonstrated a clear ability to reduce some of the mental and physical effects of stress.

Apart from the fact that rhodiola works on all three monoamines compared to St. John's Wort which just affects serotonin, rhodiola has another advantage – it doesn't interact with other medications in the same way that St. John's Wort does. So if you are taking other medication and your doctor confirms that St. John's Wort could be a problem, give rhodiola some consideration.

Magnesium

Up until a few years ago, I had always thought that magnesium helped treat anxiety for one reason - *muscles need magnesium to relax*. They use calcium to contract and magnesium to relax, which is why magnesium deficiency is associated with muscle tightness and cramping. Also, for many years we have known about the relaxing effects of *Epsom salts* baths (Epsom salts is magnesium sulfate). To be honest, for many years I believed that Epsom salts were just placebo - that people were just getting relaxed by having a hot bath. Then I read a study that appeared to demonstrate that a large amount of magnesium is absorbed through the skin when we take an Epsom salts bath. This is now known as transdermal magnesium therapy and can be extremely effective in certain situations where oral magnesium is not recommended. There is also a growing minority of health professionals who believe that transdermal therapy is a much more effective way to treat a magnesium deficiency than taking oral supplements.

Originally I thought that magnesium helped anxiety because it aided in physical relaxation. As anyone who suffers anxiety will know, there is a feedback loop that occurs between anxious thoughts and physical sensations of anxiety. By breaking that feedback loop with magnesium, anxiety can dissipate. However, recently research has emerged showing a strong correlation between magnesium levels and serotonin levels. Low magnesium is now clearly linked with low serotonin. Not only this, but a certain study also concluded that for certain patients, magnesium therapy was as effective as antidepressant medication!

New research is showing that magnesium is involved in a range of vital functions in the brain at the cellular level. Importantly, magnesium is a key co-factor in the production of serotonin, along with other vitamins such as folate and B6.

Increasingly, magnesium is being identified as a relatively potent serotonin-booster; particularly during periods of high stress (which deplete magnesium).

In the space of 2-3 short years I have witnessed an explosion of interest in magnesium for its calming, gently antidepressant qualities. I often hear from readers who have specific requests on future topics for my series of digest-form short guides. After a rather sudden spike in magnesium-related requests, I collated everything I could find to produce a quick guide on magnesium in the context of brain health, via its anxiolytic activity. This threw up some surprises, both in terms of what I was able to learn and also the popularity of this guide, which is now one of my most popular publications. One of the reasons why I write books is to distil a lot of information down to its practical and actionable essence, before the general population has caught on. However, it seems that with each passing month, more and more people are indeed catching on to the benefits of this miraculous miracle.

Curcumin (curcuma longa)

As those who have read any of my other books know, I am crazy about curcumin. This miraculous natural phenolic substance extracted from the popular spice turmeric is being researched for everything from heart disease to Alzheimer's to depression.

Curcumin's effects on the brain are so widespread that I

could have included it in several sections of this book, however for the purposes of what this book focuses on, it is curcumin's activity as a MAOI which is of most interest. Curcumin therefore increases levels of serotonin and dopamine in the brain.

However curcumin may also indirectly increase levels of these important neurotransmitters through indirect means also. Curcumin happens to be a powerful anti-inflammatory, which is interesting in that recent research has shown a clear link between inflammation and depression. Depressed brains are often inflamed brains, so cooling things off somewhat is believed to lie behind one of the reasons why curcumin acts as an antidepressant. By normalizing the inflammatory process, it is likely that serotonin levels can also normalize, however the link between serotonin and inflammation is still murky. For example, SSRIs also act as anti-inflammatories in some people and this may be one of the reasons they work to treat depression.

Curcumin also indirectly helps normalizing serotonin levels by increasing levels of BDNF (brain derived neurotrophic factor), your brain's "fertilizer". Increasing levels of BDNF theoretically accelerates the healing process, which would include your serotonergic system.

Like I said – curcumin is wonderful stuff.

However, just to reiterate (and sorry if I am starting to sound like a broken record), curcumin is appropriate for mild to moderate depression and would most likely be ineffective for more severe cases.

Kanna (Sceletium tortuosum)

Kanna is an African succulent with a long history of use by shamanistic and ethnobotanist types due to its mind-altering properties. Kanna contains a range of bioactive alkaloids including mesembrine, mesembrenol and tortuosamine which appear to boost levels of serotonin and dopamine. What makes kanna unique is that it is one of the only plant-based sources identified with clear SSRI-like behavior (e.g. - St. John's Wort appears to be closer to a MAOI, for example). Based on early promise (it has a long history of traditional use, but has only recently begun receiving research attention), Kanna is expected to becoming more widely used by the general population. At the moment, its use is restricted to those in the shaman/ethnobotanical community and those in the know. As with any herbal antidepressants, don't combine with pharmaceutical antidepressants like SSRIs.

5-htp (5-hydroxytryptophan)

5-htp is the immediate amino acid precursor to serotonin, so it makes easy intuitive sense that supplementing the building blocks of serotonin will boost serotonin. Unfortunately, reality doesn't quite match this intuitive appeal, with research studies showing inconclusive results as to whether 5-htp could be considered as a genuine natural antidepressant option. However I think this is quite expected when you consider that depression in not only involves a range of different neurotransmitters and receptors. For that matter, it is even inconclusive as to whether depression or anxiety are "caused" by low levels of neurotransmitters, and even *if* serotonin is to blame, you would then need to establish which aspect of serotonergic function is responsible. There may be an issue with receptor function, the number of receptors or a range of other serotonin-related problems. If you have an issue with either the precursor to 5-htp (the amino acid *tryptophan*) or the conversion of dietary tryptophan to serotonin, 5-htp could be immensely helpful.

5-htp is undoubtedly bioactive, as users of the drug MDMA ("ecstasy") tend to report that 5-htp markedly reduces the time it takes to recover, which is a useful piece of anecdotal information, considering the fact that MDMA boosts mood by acting as a releasing agent, forcing your brain to "dump" its supplies of serotonin into the synapse. Thus, exhausted of both serotonin and endogenous 5-htp, a 2-3 day mini-depression results.

MDMA is an interesting drug as it highlights the role played by neurotransmitters in mood. Anyone who denies that neurotransmitters like serotonin play no role in depression must account for MDMA.

This is probably a good opportunity to point out a couple of things. Firstly, rather than consigning recreational drugs to a place "over there" in any discussion of neurotransmitters and mood disorders, they should form part of the discussion if we truly wish to better understand this area. Sometimes it is the extreme examples of something which help understand the commonplace examples. Recreational drugs often involve the modulation of neurochemistry far beyond what is typical. For example, certain things like social interaction, empathetic thoughts or a feeling of total safety, give your brain a little squirt from the "serotonin bottle". MDMA says *screw this!* and unscrews the lid, pouring serotonin into the brain. So by understanding what MDMA (or cocaine et al.) does to the brain and how this correlates with subjective or behavioral effects, tells us quite a bit about the role the various neurotransmitters play in mood or behavior.

Secondly, it literally pains me to write the word "anecdotal", as I am cognizant of how much weight science places on anecdotes versus properly-designed, placebo-controlled studies. However my view is that, whilst anecdotes should never be used in isolation to make judgements, they can provide a useful source of information to support more scientific data.

In addition, it is often anecdotes which first highlight something that can then be studied scientifically. If we look back over the past century, many of the things we now know to be toxic, were once considered benign. In each case, it is the initial accumulation of anecdotal health reports which then led to proper analysis. For example, in the early 20th century, young ladies worked in factories painting watch dials with radium-laced paint to give it enough glow for soldiers to check the time without revealing themselves to the enemy. It wasn't until authorities noticed these ladies dying in huge numbers that they decide to investigate scientifically. When the bones of the victims were placed on the film used to make x-rays and left overnight, when they checked the film in the morning, the bones were so radioactive that they imprinted an impression on the film. Hence the combination of anecdote (as an initial signaling mechanism) with scientific rigor (to confirm or refute the anecdote) led to an advancement of understanding.

5-htp is well and truly at the anecdote stage. There has been some scientific study already, however the results are generally mixed at best. Yet there are *anecdotes* of people finding 5-htp to be the single most effective antidepressant they have used. You could potentially be one of these people, so a trial of 5-htp could potentially be an option if this is suspected.

Cognitive & behavioral therapy (CBT)

If you have never received psychotherapy before, you probably imagine a scenario involving old-school psychoanalysis, where a therapist asks you various Freudian questions, probing your relationship with your mother, all the while reclining on a sofa while the therapist listens with apparent disinterest. Fortunately this is largely a thing of the past, replaced with modern, scientific therapies like CBT. I am not a trained cognitive behavioral therapist and in any case, there are already plenty of great books available on this topic, written by professional therapists. (Feeling Good: The New Mood Therapy by David

Burns is a good place to start.) However, essentially CBT involves the identification and remediation of faulty thinking and behavior which contributes to depression and anxiety. Have you ever been in a good mood, only to think of something upsetting or stressful, only to see your mood dive? Have you ever noticed how certain behaviors put you in a good mood whereas other behaviors do the opposite? That is essentially the principle which underpins CBT.

Mood disorders like depression are typically associated with distortions in thought patterns ("I am worthless", "I will never feel good again", "If this presentation goes badly it will be a disaster" and so on.) Over time, negative thinking and behavior will drive down serotonin levels. Only in a minority of cases is depression caused simply by a biological issue like low serotonin. More common, an event or a serious of (usually stressful) events pushes down serotonin levels, with depression resulting. However this misses a key step, which is where CBT comes in. It is not actually the events per se, but the thinking that follows. How would you feel if you left your car in a car park, only to return and find it on fire, a burnt out shell? Pretty bad right? What about if you hated the car and it was insured for more than its current value? As you can see, it is not events per se, but our relationship to them. CBT involves the gradual identification of any thoughts and behaviors which are keeping your mood down or anxiety levels up.

Over time, CBT is associated with the same neurological

changes that drug therapy is known for, such as increased hippocampal volume (People with depression often have shrunken hippocampi) and is associated with serotonergic activity normalizing. Compared to those who take antidepressants only, people who also received CBT tend to relapse into depression at much lesser rates, suggesting enduring pro-serotonin effects.

Another reason why CBT is powerfully effective at increasing serotonin levels is the subject of the next section.

Sense of Control

There is a very famous rodent experiment that I often tell people about as it is a powerful representation of an important fact regarding serotonin (and general well-being) that most people have never heard of. If you put a mouse in an environment where it receives electric shocks but is able to escape to a safe area or platform, they tend to cope OK. However if you put the same mouse in a situation where it is receiving electric shocks yet has no means of escape, soon the mouse starts exhibiting signs of depression! Post mortem tests on these rodents also show clearly reduce serotonin levels or changes in receptor density.

The human equivalent is the dead end job, the abusive relationship or any other way a person can lose the sense that they are "in control". Many therapists have observed the phenomenon where people can actually handle a large degree of adversity and stress, in general coping adequately. However once someone feels things are out of control or beyond their control, depression and anxiety disorders often result.

The prescription here is clear – Take charge of your life. Particularly regarding things which are affecting your mental well-being. Even sitting down to make a plan on how to rectify your situation will send dopamine and serotonin levels dramatically higher. Go ahead and try it. Identify something in your life that you would like to regain control over. Sit down and write down a plan on how you are going to remedy this situation. I think you will be blown away by the results. In the planning and execution stage, the dopamine boost will be more obvious, however once you have achieved your goal and the dopamine spurt slows down you will find that gradually serotonin levels will rise.

Meditation

So if we clearly understand that stress depletes not only serotonin, but many other key neurotransmitters, surely a logical question to ask is – *What is the opposite to stress?* Surely deep relaxation and a worry-free state will boost serotonin. The good news is that not only does deep relaxation boost serotonin, we have access to possibly the single most powerful relaxation tool and it is completely free (Unless you pay one of those ridiculous places to receive a "special mantra").

Meditation is one of the most powerful brain tonics available, causing a range of powerful *neurotrophic* (the opposite to *neurotoxic*) effects. I usually defer to Benjamin Kramer regarding the effects of meditation and the brain. In his (somewhat unimaginatively-titled) book *Meditation and the Brain*, Kramer gathered a ton of research on the topic -

Researchers reported that meditation also has a huge range of physiological benefits. These benefits include increased cardiac output, muscle relaxation, elevated serotonin and melatonin levels along with noteworthy improvements in chronic pain. Cardiac output refers to the amount of blood pumped by the heart. The more blood being pumped by the heart, the more oxygen and nutrients the body receives. Serotonin is a chemical derived from the amino acid tryptophan which is one of the primary neurotransmitters involved in emotional function (most antidepressants work at least in part by increasing levels of serotonin). Melatonin is a hormone derived from serotonin and secreted by the pineal gland, which produces changes in the skin color of vertebrates, reptiles, and amphibians, and is essential in regulating biorhythms. You may have seen melatonin being sold as a supplement for improving sleep or treating jetlag.

Even though I am a passionate meditator, I am no meditation teacher and this is no specialist meditation book. I am the last person qualified to be espousing any one technique or, god forbid, handing out unsolicited spiritual advice. If you are interested, I heartily recommend you check out one of the many books available on this topic. Some of the authors I consider to be authentic, true experts in their field are:

- Jon Kabat-Zinn
- Thich Nhat Hanh
- Ram Dass
- Adyashanti
- Matthieu Riccard

Each of these authors bring a unique perspective, be it mindfulness, Zen Buddhism or a more general flavor.

However, as a small entrée into this sprawling topic, let me provide a couple of examples.

A simple "breath" meditation

In his book *Meditation and the Brain*, Benjamin Kramer provided a nice and simple example of how to meditate on the breath. He has kindly allowed me to reproduce the instructions here:

1) *Sit up in a comfortable position*
2) *Take a few deep, slow breaths and concentrate on the sensation of air passing through your nostrils*
3) *Count "one" on the 'in-breath' and "two" on the 'out-breath' all the way to "10" and then start again at "one".*
4) *When you find your thoughts wandering, just start again at "one". A useful way to notice that your mind has wandered is when you say "eleven" – that's your sign to tell you that you have passed "ten" because you were thinking about something else.*

5) *When your mind wanders (and it WILL wander), just bring it back to "one" and don't get frustrated. This is the number one mistake that beginners make. They think that the purpose of meditation is to completely stop thinking. This is impossible and is not the goal of meditation. The act of realizing your mind has wandered and then bringing it back to your breath - that is meditation.*

6) *If you do this prior to bed, after a little while you will struggle to stay awake, so just lay down and enjoy the relaxed feeling. You will soon drop off to sleep.*

However I also want to point out that meditation doesn't have the monopoly on relaxation techniques. In fact, if you are currently depressed or suffering from an anxiety disorder, there is a school of thought that says you should avoid meditation and focus on more physical relaxation techniques until you get better. Meditation involves bringing your thoughts into clear focus and for someone agitated or disturbed, this can sometimes be counterproductive. This is where activities such as Tai Chi, Yoga or even gardening can be helpful.

Don't get stuck on a single path up the mountain. Find out what works for you. There are countless relaxation techniques, from biofeedback to binaural beats to progressive muscle relaxation. Don't be afraid to experiment to find the technique that works for you.

Your serotonin receptors with thank you for it.

Loving-kindness

One of the most powerful Buddhist meditation techniques (which has correlates in many other religions including Christianity) is the loving-kindness meditation, which involves filling your mind with loving thoughts directed at those around you, all living creatures and even the entire universe. Naturally there are a range of metaphysical explanations for why exactly this is such a powerful technique for increasing well-being, however from my perspective I am interested in the potent serotonin-boosting effects.

Again, this is easy to verify with a simple experiment. Spend 5-10 minutes thinking about the people you hate, why you hate them (or, if you don't hate anyone, people that annoy you or you dislike). Take a moment to look at your mind-set and physiology. These kinds of thoughts are associated with muscle tension, increased heart rate and *dysphoria* (the opposite of *euphoria*). Now spend the same amount of time thinking about those you love and why you love them. An extremely powerful element of this meditation is thinking about the people you hate or dislike, but trying to view the world from their perspective. Remember, just like you, they were born a small helpless child and have gone through various tough experiences which have shaped how they are today.

Socialize

As I detailed in *The Methuselah Project*, one of the most

powerful predictors of long life is socialization. Amongst all the longest-lived people in the world, such as those in the small villages of Okinawa, Japan, to their counterparts in Sardinia, Italy, one of the key unifying factors is that they also possess strong community bonds.

As you may have noticed, a key way of looking at serotonin is – What are the things we do or think when we are depressed? Do the opposite.

One of the most reliable indicators of depression is isolation. Depression causes people to isolate themselves and isolation in turn, causes depression. And very often, just like sparks and fires, where there is depression, there is often low serotonin lurking. Serotonin is innately linked to home mammals socialize. Alpha male gorillas have high serotonin and submissive gorillas with no power or mating privileges have low serotonin. The human correlate to this is the corporate world with the energetic, resilient CEO and the unhappy bottom-rung drones.

One way to break this vicious cycle is to force yourself to socialize and form stronger bonds with those around you. Reconnect with old friends and distant relatives. Join community groups. Whatever it takes to get you reconnected. You will be astounded at the effects – I promise.

Oh, and if you want to really turbo-charge this process, join a volunteer organization helping those less fortunate than you. This combines two powerful antidepressants in one – social connection and self-esteem. If helping others was a drug, it would be a blockbuster.

Boosting serotonin is quite simple and logical. Avoid the things that make you feel bad and do the things that make you feel good. Anything relaxing and enjoyable will usually boost serotonin. Massage? Yep. Getting out in the sunshine? You betcha. Draw up a list of things you like doing and the things you need to remove from your life. The improvement can be dramatic.

Oh, and one piece of bad news to finish on. This is so important that I wanted to leave you with it. Alcohol is probably the most common serotonin-killer in modern society. Not only does alcohol send serotonin levels lower after the initial high, it keeps you from entering into the deep sleep stage where your serotonin levels are usually replaced. If you think you may have low serotonin, sorry however you will need to either cut it out completely for a while or at least cut back to levels that won't cause you problems.

Dopamine

Happy, motivated, confident & energized

Considering how important dopamine is, our knowledge of exactly what it does in our brains is surprisingly imprecise. As you may have read, dopamine is a *catecholamine* neurotransmitter, which, along with noradrenaline and glutamate, is one of your main *excitatory* neurotransmitters.

You have probably read that dopamine is your "pleasure", "motivation" and "reward" neurotransmitter and that when your brain squirts dopamine it feels great. As usual, reality is a little more complicated.

Our understanding for some time now has been that, when you obtain something important (from an evolutionary perspective) such as food or sexual gratification, your brain releases a pleasurable rush of dopamine to make you feel "good" and thereby encouraging you to repeat the activity. This is why addictive disorders have always been associated with dopaminergic dysfunction, causing people to seek out the same particular thing (such as a drug) over and over. This is considered a dysfunction because it is not hard to imagine the problems that addictive disorders would have created for our distant ancestors.

However recent research published in the journal *Neuron* casts some doubt over this simplified understanding. Joint Spanish and American study found that it is also dopamine that drives you to seek out these rewards in the first place. Not only this, they also found that persistence is likely linked to high dopamine, so the higher the dopamine levels, the more you are likely to soldier on through adversity to achieve a particular goal.

One of the most interesting aspects of dopamine however is how it mediates both psychological motivation (towards a goal or reward) and the actual physical movement which carries you towards whatever the goal happens to be. The part of the brain that is responsible for this, the *basal ganglia*, is largely controlled by dopamine. If you look at a glass of water and decide to pick it up and drink it because you are thirsty, it is dopamine (via the basal ganglia) which controls the initiation of movement which takes your hand to the glass to pick it up. This is why, when the dopamine-producing neurons in a part of the basal ganglia known as the *substantia nigra* are destroyed, Parkinson's disease is similar disorders is the result.

I bet you thought things couldn't get more complicated regarding dopamine right? In recent years the situation has become further clouded by the concept of *reward prediction error*. Scientists conducting rodent experiments have found that the dopaminergic system is even more complicated than we thought. The classical understanding of dopamine is that an animal sees food (or a potential mate) and consequently experiences a pleasurable burst of dopamine to encourage them to see out the reward and then do something similar again in the future.

However there is a problem with this that you may know from personal experience. Imagine you are walking down the street and you notice an ice cream store has opened so you go inside and order the most delicious ice cream you have ever tasted. How good is that feeling? Next time you know that you will need to pass by that ice cream store you will get a little jolt of dopaminergic pleasure thinking about getting one of those great ice creams again. But we all know how this story ends. By the fifth or tenth time (or sooner in some cases), you have grown accustomed to getting that ice cream and you no longer get much pleasure from it. In fact, if you check your mind-state closely, you may find that you *thought* you were getting pleasure but were really just chasing a kind of ephemeral pleasure just out of reach and were simply acting out of habit.

Unfortunately, dopamine is a *"MORE! MORE! MORE!"* neurotransmitter and is never happy with the same thing over and over. You need to keep chasing that bigger and better pleasure. Dopamine loves novelty, which is why travel can give us so much pleasure. Put another way, if something (like ice cream) is abundant, the parts of your brain responsible for reward and reinforcement (which use dopamine to signal) lose interest as they assume that they don't need to ensure you take advantage of it because it isn't as rare as first thought.

This understanding underpins the concept of reward prediction error and has thrown up interesting results in animal trials. Researchers found that, when a mouse experienced the same reward more than once, dopamine wasn't just automatically released when the mouse saw the reward again. Dopamine levels only rose if the reward was greater than expected and if the reward was less than expected, dopamine levels dropped.

I call this the *pay rise phenomenon*. If you are expecting a $10,000 pay rise and you only get $5000 you would feel terrible wouldn't you? Your brain (and your dopamine!) doesn't care that a $5000 increase is more than you were previously earning. It only compares your expectation with reality and if reality doesn't match expectation, dopamine levels drop and you feel displeasure.

So, in summary, dopamine likes new things, rare things and pleasant surprises.

The parts of the brain which are chiefly run by dopamine are the basal ganglia (which you already know about), the nucleus accumbens (which is part of the basal ganglia, to be specific) and the ventral tegmental area (VTA). I want to avoid focusing on individual brain structures too much because this is not a neurology book and also when we look at structures of the brain we can disappear down a rabbit hole that doesn't get us any closer to understanding how our mind works. However in some cases, specific mention of particular brain structures can be instructive.

The symptoms of low dopamine activity

The symptoms of low dopamine are, in general, reasonably unsurprising when you think of it as your energy/mood/pleasure neurotransmitter, however there are one or two symptoms which are less obvious –

- **Hypersomnia (too much sleep) and difficulty getting out of bed in the morning -** By the way, please don't diagnose yourself as having low dopamine based on this alone. Not having a spring in your step when you wake up would probably describe 99% of the adult population! However if this is a chronic problem for you, dopamine may be involved.

- **Lack of ability to feel pleasure from the things that normally interest you (*anhedonia*) -** This is also a tricky one to diagnose because the concept of "pleasure" is ill-defined. In my case, I have come to understand periods where I am anhedonic, but this is only after considerable introspection. In my case, these (brief) periods are characterized by a lack of that excited feeling you get in your tummy when you do something you enjoy or hear good news. It is also difficult to clearly differentiate between "pleasure" and "happiness". Can you tell the difference? This is one of the reasons why people sometimes get confused when they hear both serotonin *and* dopamine referred to as "the feel-good neurotransmitter". In general, serotonin is a more contented, relaxed kind of positive mood whereas dopamine is a more excited, motivated and (sometimes) euphoric kind of positive mood.

- **Lack of motivation** - For me, this is reflected in less planning of new projects, with more time spent aimlessly surfing the net or watching TV. This does not mean that surfing the net or watching TV means you are low in dopamine. It is more about the mind state that underpins activities like these. If you want to unwind in front of the TV after a long hard day or take a time out to surf the net, it doesn't mean that there is anything wrong. However if you find yourself procrastinating or lacking the spark to work on the projects you normally enjoy, this could be an indication of a dopamine related problem.

- **Depression** - Severely low dopamine can also cause a kind of low motivation/lack of pleasure/apathetic depression. As mentioned in the FAQ, serotonin depression and dopamine depression are distinctly different. I have usually found that dopamine related depression tends to lack the anxiety component that serotonin depression does.

- **More introverted than usual** -Dopamine gives you confidence, so out of character introversion could suggest an issue with this neurotransmitter. However even this point is tricky when trying to differentiate between serotonin related introversion and dopamine related introversion. Low serotonin is associated with a lack of social power (Dominant primates tend to have higher levels of serotonin) which can also manifest with a kind of introversion. Therefore, only use introversion as one of several symptoms to point towards dopamine being a problem as introversion alone is not reliable enough.

- **Lack of mental energy** - Low dopamine can also cause you to mentally fatigue earlier than usual. This lack of mental energy can also manifest via a lack of concentration.

- **Weight gain** - It is unclear why low dopamine is associated with weight gain however I believe it is linked to both the low energy problem and also changes to hormonal signaling. Drugs that boost dopamine (like cocaine and methamphetamine) cause weight loss due to the fact that they keep your motor revving higher and suppress appetite, so logically the opposite must also be true.

- **Need caffeine to get a boost** - Caffeine (among other things) gives your dopamine a modest boost. This is why a coffee lover will get an unusually strong mood boost just thinking about having a cup of coffee. This is also why, under reward prediction error, that second cup of coffee is never as good. For coffee addicts, dopamine hijacks your brain and tells you I MUST GET COFFEE NOW!

- **Addictive personality -** As mentioned earlier, addictions and dopamine go hand in hand. When you become addicted to something, dopamine teams up with glutamate to hijack your brain and tell you that you must keep doing whatever it is you are addicted to. Addictions can include anything related to your reward and pleasure center (you nucleus accumbens in particular) such as drugs or sex. Addictive behavior can therefore sometimes be viewed as your brain's attempt to get more dopamine.

- **Reduced sex drive -** Your libido is strongly linked to dopamine. No dopamine – no desire to have sex. There is also a close relationship between dopamine and testosterone, so if you are suffering from low sex drive (whether you are male or female, surprisingly), testosterone could possibly also be the culprit.

How to boost levels of dopamine

If you believe that you are suffering from low dopamine and wish to remedy this, there is good news and bad news. The good news is that dopamine is relatively easy to boost via drug and non-drug means. The bad news is that, because dopamine is central to your reward system, increasing dopamine via pharmaceuticals is fraught with addiction risk and tolerance problems. If you discover a way to boost dopamine, your brain will force you, with some degree of urgency, to do whatever is was, over and over. Then, as tolerance takes hold, you will need larger and larger doses to achieve the same effect. This is contrasted with serotonin, which is not typically associated with tolerance and addiction. This is a potential explanation for why methamphetamine (which works mainly on dopamine and noradrenaline) is highly addictive, yet the closely related MDMA (ecstasy), which works predominantly on serotonin and much lesser so on dopamine, is not considered addictive.

My general feeling when it comes to boosting dopamine is to first exhaust all non-drug options before you consider the pharmaceutical route. I believe that dopamine is much more responsive to certain behaviors and thought processes than serotonin is – at least in the short term, as therapies like CBT can, over time, also boost serotonin.

Pharmaceutical options

In general, if you wish to boost dopamine via pharmaceuticals, you are looking at the stimulant class of drugs, as boosting dopamine gives you energy and usually involves a similar rise in noradrenaline. And, assuming you are not suicidal/moronic and have wisely decided to avoid street drugs such as meth and cocaine to achieve this, your options are

75

essentially the two main medications used to treat ADD/ADHD – methylphenidate (Ritalin) and dextroamphetamine (or as Adderall, which is a mixture of dextroamphetamine and levoamphetamine).

Methylphenidate (Ritalin)

Methylphenidate is a dopamine reuptake inhibitor used to treat ADD and ADHD, along with a variety of off-label uses for people suffering from either extreme tiredness (due to narcolepsy or sleep apnea) or dopamine related depression.

Methylphenidate has always been the subject of considerable controversy due to the fact that it works in a similar way to cocaine, albeit at much lesser potency and addictiveness. Whilst this is technically true, just because one drug works in a similar fashion to an illegal drug, it doesn't make it necessarily "bad". The codeine you take for pain works the same way as heroin. The painkiller tramadol is a serotonin releasing agent just like MDMA (ecstasy).

I boil it down to this – If you are suffering from severe and chronic dopamine related problems, methylphenidate can be a miracle drug that literally saves your life. If your deficiency is more subtle and less disabling, stay away from stimulants and focus on gentler options.

Dextroamphetamine[5] (and levoamphetamine)

Your other legal stimulant option is amphetamine, which is the other main medication used to treat disorders related to attention and focus. While both methylphenidate and dextroamphetamine increase levels of dopamine, the latter is much less targeted on dopamine. Amphetamine essentially triggers the release of your brain's stores of dopamine, norepinephrine and, to a much lesser extent, serotonin.

If you have both low dopamine and low norepinephrine, amphetamines would be a potent option. However if you have a dopamine specific problem or are at the milder end of the spectrum, give them a miss. Research also appears to indicate that the addiction risk with amphetamine is higher than with methylphenidate.

Roughly speaking, the main difference between the dextro and levo forms is that dextroamphetamine tends to be more mood boosting, whereas levoamphetamine tends to be more energizing physically.

Nicotine

As mentioned in the update at the beginning of this book, I have spent a good deal of time recently studying the pharmacology of nicotine, based on an emerging body of research which is painting an altogether more nuanced picture of

---

[5] Often shortened to dexamphetamine or colloquially, *dexies*.

this much maligned drug. I should point out that my opinion of tobacco and of cigarette smoking remains unchanged. Cigarettes are possibly one of the most evil inventions of man imaginable. According to the World Health Organization, more than 6 million people die each year from smoking-related causes.

However, when we separate nicotine (which is only one of the many bioactive substances found in tobacco) from tobacco, a slightly more nuanced picture emerges.

As part of my research into this drug, I have discovered that there are a large number of people using nicotine patches and gums, despite having never smoked a single cigarette in their life. Why are they doing this?

Nicotine exerts its effects on the brain primarily by activating *nicotinic acetylcholine receptors* (which, I should point out, are named after nicotine, not the other way around). Firstly, this boosts cholinergic neurotransmission, one of the neurochemical foundations required for your brain to learn and retain new information or skills. However, one of the indirect effects of this is increased levels of dopamine. As increased levels of cholinergic and dopaminergic activity are two of the most powerful routes to accelerated brain function, it is not surprising that many have looked towards nicotine as a brain enhancer. Recently, this dopamine-boosting quality possessed by nicotine has even seen it being studied in those with depression caused by low dopamine. Imagine that discussion between the researchers and the potential test subjects! ("You want me to take *what* for depression?").

In the interests of being able to talk from at least some position of experience, for the benefit of you, my trusty reader, I have trialed nicotine gum for a few days. I should point out that I have never ingested nicotine[6], so could be considered nicotine naïve in terms of tolerance. The first time I tried nicotine gum, I neglected to properly read the instructions and chewed the gum like it was normal chewing gum (For those non-smokers out there – nicotine gum is supposed to be chewed briefly before being "parked" in your gums, which slowly absorb the nicotine). Clearly I received a dose of nicotine which was much higher than I had envisaged and promptly became lightheaded, dizzy and a little bit high. Despite this, I can't say that I would describe the experience as unequivocally pleasant, rather, it felt like I was cycling rapidly between pleasant and unpleasant. However this was likely a function of the dose. Subsequent attempts (using the correct ingestion method) resulted in an altogether more subtle effect involving slightly increased energy levels.

Unfortunately I have so far been unable to reliably generate either improved mood or substantially improved cognitive abilities. However I should point out that one person (me) isn't statistically significant and also I am not depressed or even low in

---

[6] Actually this is not strictly true. Upon reflection, I probably smoked multiple packs of cigarettes passively when I was a child, thanks to the various adults who were considerate enough to smoke in close proximity to me.

dopamine (that I know of).

So if I could summarize my experience with nicotine (both practical and theoretical), it would be that it shows great theoretical promise for situations where low dopamine may be an issue, however in my case I haven't really seen enough tangible evidence that would encourage me to consider nicotine as an ongoing option for me personally, as either a learning aid or just a nice "pick me up".

However if there is one key piece of knowledge I have emerged with based on my reading of the research it is that nicotine's addictiveness (something most would consider beyond question) is supported by relatively weak evidence. For example, no sane person would ever question the addictiveness of tobacco, however in trials looking at the addictiveness of pure nicotine, either in humans or animals, there appears to be very little evidence that nicotine is actually the addictive part of tobacco. For example, the pleasant experience felt by cigarette smokers has been linked to substances in tobacco which act as MAOIs – yes the same MAOI action seen in old-school antidepressants.

I should point out however that the topic of nicotine's addictiveness is far from decided, just that there is evidence either way. I am sure many smokers reading this book may point to their inability to eventually give up nicotine patches or gum. However in pure statistical terms, studies looking at this topic have tended to find that nicotine is at best only weakly addictive.

I tend to think that different people will respond differently, depending on how they are wired and their environment (stress levels etc.), so the issue of addictiveness should at least be given some consideration by any previous non-smoker considering using nicotine to boost dopamine.

Natural and drug-free ways to boost dopamine

So, would you like to now hear the good news?

Dopamine is amazingly malleable through engaging in particular activities and dopamine-promoting thinking habits. There is a two way relationship between dopamine and your thoughts. Boosting dopamine gives you optimism, energy, motivation and confidence. Likewise, by engaging in motivating or rewarding activities, you boost your dopamine.

There is a fantastic research paper by neuroscientist Kelly Lambert which is essentially unknown outside of very specific scientific circles. This is a shame because this particular paper is fascinating and introduces a novel concept in the field of mood disorders. Lambert puts forward the term *effort-based rewards* to explain the apparent rise in depression across the world as humans have gradually moved away from our traditional, pre-industrial revolution life.

In the distant past, humans had a more direct link between their actions and rewarding outcomes. They would need to bring down a bison or catch rabbits with their own hands. This is a simple reward that your dopamine system is set up for. You do something and it leads to a reward. However now, this has been replaced, in many cases, by a simple trip to your refrigerator to extract food without any effort. Lambert hypothesizes that this lack of stereotypical dopamine-promoting activities may be behind many cases of depression across the globe.

So logically, the way to short-circuit this process is to engage in activities (effort) which lead to a rewarding outcome. Have you ever wondered why it feels so great to look at your freshly spring-cleaned house or washed car? That feeling is the concept of effort-based rewards at work. So, if you want to keep dopamine levels high, even if you don't feel like it, do something effortful and difficult which leads to a rewarding outcome. For me, it's writing books. Nothing beats that intense dopamine surge I get when I publish a new book. Your path may be different.

I also believe this is a major reason why CBT is so effective at relieving depression. Not only does CBT boost serotonin, it also boosts dopamine due to the effort-based rewards principle. CBT is very goal-oriented, involving the setting of a range of short and medium term goals as part of your therapy. Setting (and achieving) goals is one of the most powerful ways to boost dopamine that we know of.

So what kinds of activities could this include? In theory, anything that gives you reward for effort will do. So this could be –

- **Write a book** – Of course, I am biased, however have you ever thought about writing a book? With Amazon's KDP program, once you have written your book, all you need is a simple cover and to write a blurb before you can go live across the world. Would seeing your book for sale on Amazon give you a dopamine surge?

- **Home projects** – DIY or renovation projects are perfect activities for increasing dopamine because you can see and enjoy a tangible outcome. There is nothing abstract about a new outdoor BBQ area or a freshly painted house. Dopamine loves this kind of thing!

These are just a couple of ideas. There are literally thousands of different things you could do to boost dopamine in this way. Your brain loves planning, so it gives you a nice squirt of dopamine when you make plans to improve your situation, change things for the better or in some way do something which will be beneficial for you. Evolutionarily speaking, planning signifies survival, so it makes sense that your brain rewards you by jacking up dopamine levels. The plan doesn't even have to come to fruition. Just making the plan and resolving to execute it is sufficient.

Interestingly, Lambert also identifies a specific type of activity which appears to be more powerful than anything else – using your hands! Out brain dedicates a disproportionately large amount of area for controlling and sensing (touch) through your hands. Your hands, with their trusty opposable thumbs, are one of the key factors behind the success of humans as a species. So, if you want to really turbo-charge your dopamine levels, create things with your hands. The most obvious ways to use your hands to create is via hobbies like woodworking, knitting, pottery and even making model airplanes. However I think that the activity you choose must involve conscious focus on the hands. Mouse clicks won't cut it.

So, thinking about sex triggers dopamine and so does using your hands. Perhaps this explains the second favorite habit of male humans?

In terms of supplements, there are a few options. Firstly, you can try L-tyrosine or L-phenylalanine supplements, which provide the building blocks for dopamine (and noradrenaline). However this will only work if this is the reason why your dopamine is low. For many people, their dopamine levels are low for other reasons, so if you have no problems with consuming enough tyrosine-rich protein or converting tyrosine to dopamine, supplementing with tyrosine or phenylalanine is unlikely to do much. Another option is the herb mucuna pruriens, which contains high levels of L-DOPA, the immediate precursor to dopamine. Mucuna pruriens can be so successful that it is even used by some Parkinson's disease patients to relieve some of the symptoms of the disease.

Another, much weaker, way to increase dopamine is by using a herbal monoamine oxidase inhibitor, such as rhodiola rosea or curcumin, both of which I am very fond of as gentle antidepressants.

Noradrenaline

Dopamine's energizing half-sister

First things first. You may have been confused by the use of the terms *noradrenaline* and *norepinephrine* interchangeably. They are the same thing, however noradrenaline (which is used in most parts of the world) is derived from Latin and norepinephrine (which is used in the USA, thanks to the US National Library of Medicine, for reasons I have never bothered looking up[7]) is derived from Greek. If you are wondering why I

---

[7] Edit – OK I thought this seemed half-assed so I went and looked it up. Apparently a pharmaceutical company had an adrenaline product called, conveniently, Adrenalin, so it was decided to switch the generic name to avoid confusion. Fun Fact of the day.

generally stick to noradrenaline, my reasoning is surprisingly prosaic – the word norepinephrine is really, really annoying to touch type. Go ahead[8] – try it!

Also, the difference between adrenaline and noradrenaline is also complicated, however in general, think of noradrenaline as being a neurotransmitter released by and acting on parts of your brain, with adrenaline being distributed around your body to prepare you for "fight or flight".

Noradrenaline is very closely related to dopamine and they are both synthesized by the same amino acid – L-tyrosine. If you stimulate the release of noradrenaline only (and not dopamine), the result is typically just stimulation (rapid heartbeat, increased body temperature, increased alertness). However if you trigger the release of noradrenaline and dopamine at the same, you get a degree of euphoria much more potent than if you released dopamine only. There is a strong synergistic effect when you add in energy to a euphoric brain. This is why pure noradrenaline re-uptake inhibitors (like the ghastly and generally ineffective reboxetine) tend to have a poor ability to improve mood.

However that's not to say that noradrenaline is unrelated to mood whatsoever. Energy can boost mood. However there is a difference between something being euphoric and something improving mood a little. In general though, noradrenaline works better in combination with other neurotransmitters. This is why the older classes of antidepressants (monoamine oxidase inhibitors and tricyclic antidepressants) are actually more effective than the SSRI's (which work primarily on serotonin) common today. However the addition of noradrenaline into the equation is also the main reason these older drugs aren't used any more, as tweaking noradrenaline creates a range of side-effects ranging from annoying (like orthostatic hypotension, where you get dizzy when you stand up) to life-threatening (If you take an overdose of tricyclics like amitriptyline you can actually die, as they are cardiotoxic in higher doses). Fortunately there are some newer drugs like duloxetine and venlafaxine which boost noradrenaline and serotonin but don't create overdose or toxicity risk.

Another way to explain noradrenaline's importance in mood disorders is to think in terms of someone who is depressed and lethargic, with barely enough energy to get out of bed. If you can give noradrenaline a boost, it can act like a jump-start, enabling the person to start recommencing some of the activities that can, in turn, trigger pleasure. However generally, if you give a noradrenaline boost to someone functioning normally, with normal energy levels, there is unlikely to be much boost in mood unless dopamine is also boosted. In actual fact, what is more likely, is that by just boosting noradrenaline you risk triggering anxiety or panic, which is no fun at all.

There is a reason why stimulants used to treat ADHD work so well – Noradrenaline is a powerful modulator of attention. This is not surprising when you think back to our evolutionary past. If your distant ancestors encountered a dangerous animal, it would be fatal if their mind drifted off and started thinking about that lovely cave painting they just finished. Your brain triggers the release of noradrenaline to tell you *"This is really important so you'd better pay attention"*.

The symptoms of low noradrenaline

The main symptoms of low noradrenaline are not particularly surprising, considering what it does. They include –

- ➢ Lack of energy
- ➢ Lack of motivation
- ➢ Lack of focus and attention
- ➢ Sleeping too much
- ➢ Depressed mood

There is a great deal of debate in psychiatry around our focus on serotonin's role in depression. As some researchers have pointed out, if someone presents in a doctor's office complaining of the above symptoms, most of the time they will walk away with a prescription for an SSRI. This is despite the apparent fact that depression caused by problems with serotonin, dopamine and noradrenaline looks quite different. If this describes your experience with your doctor, perhaps it could be a good idea to ask for options that boost noradrenaline also (apart from reboxetine, which is widely considered ineffective) or seek a second opinion.

Optimizing noradrenaline is relatively straightforward, whether via pharmaceuticals or otherwise:

Optimizing noradrenaline with pharmaceuticals

The most potent way to boost noradrenaline quickly is with amphetamines, which probably comes as no surprise. However some other options include –

Tricyclic antidepressants

These drugs tend to act on a wide range of systems in your body and brain, which is why they are often referred to as *dirty* drugs (*clean* drugs tend to have specific actions). However mainly they act as serotonin and noradrenaline re-uptake inhibitors. Each type of tricyclic has differing relative potency regarding serotonin and noradrenaline, ranging from clomipramine which mainly works on serotonin, to desipramine, which mainly works on noradrenaline.

Some of the more commonly-used tricyclics include amitriptyline, clomipramine and desipramine, however there are many more, each with their own unique traits. For example, clomipramine is primarily serotonergic, whereas desipramine and dothiepin (dosulepin) are more noradrenaline-focused. Amitryptiline is a good example of a balanced option.

Another way to classify each tricyclic is by its antihistamine properties, with tricyclics as a group tending to be fairly potent activators of your H_1 histamine receptor. Hence, many can make you sleepy, which is why they are often prescribed as hypnotics for people with sleeping issues. The downside of this however, is that, like any other first generation antihistamine, tricyclics can make you gain a considerable amount of weight.

Monoamine oxidase inhibitors (MAOIs)

These older drugs tend to extremely effective, yet comparatively dangerous because particular foods can trigger a hypertensive crisis, leading to death. If you are in a deep, dark hole and are one step away from electro-convulsive therapy (ECT), then MAOIs could be a life-saving option. If you are looking to give your neurochemicals a nice handy boost, don't even think about MAOIs. There is however a key distinction. Some natural substances (such as rhodiola rosea and curcumin) act as weak MAOIs, as does the more recent drug moclobemide. However these are known as *reversible* MAOIs and don't come with the same dangers that the older *irreversible* MAOIs do.

Natural and drug-free options for boosting noradrenaline

In general, anything that increases noradrenaline will be prescription only. The closest thing to a natural noradrenaline booster would be *ma huang*, which contains ephedrine. However ma huang really only increases adrenaline and it is illegal now in most countries.

However behaviorally, it is easy to increase noradrenaline levels temporarily – Just do things that excite you. Looking forward to something enjoyable, with a sense of excited anticipation and then the experience itself will boost levels of noradrenaline.

This is all stuff you should be doing anyway, however I would caution anyone looking to preferentially boost noradrenaline. I always suggest people focus on serotonin and dopamine because, if you get those two right, noradrenaline usually resolves also.

Be Your Own Detective

How to tell whether you are depressed (and/or anxious) due to low serotonin, dopamine or noradrenaline

It is one thing to regurgitate everything I know on this topic based on the experiences of others, however I wanted to be able to speak with at least some degree of personal experience. So, in the interests of experimentation, I have done something unusual. Through pharmacological means (which I won't go into, as I don't want anyone else "trying this at home" so to speak) I tried deliberately depleting or suppressing levels of serotonin, noradrenaline and dopamine, one by one, to see how distinct the experience was.

The results were quite startling.

Serotonin

Low serotonin has a very distinct feel to it. In my case, I experienced –

- **Anxiety** – This was the biggest difference between serotonin depressed and dopamine depressed. For me, low dopamine featured a strange absence of any anxiety, whereas low serotonin made me rather anxious.
- **Lower self-confidence** – Most noticeable in situations requiring larger groups of people.
- **Digestive problems** - For your sake I won't go into specifics, however mostly involved stomach sensitivity and cramps.
- **Poor sleep quality** – Waking up feeling tired and cranky
- **Increased irritability** (which verged on aggression at times.) Fortunately I didn't do anything regrettable, however I felt like snapping at people sometimes when they said something to annoy me. This is very unusual behavior for me.

Dopamine and Noradrenaline

Regarding dopamine and noradrenaline I will put them into the same category as it is difficult to target one and not the other.

For example, drugs that act on dopamine (such as methylphenidate) also have actions on noradrenaline and drugs that are more noradrenaline-specific (such as dexamphetamine) also act on dopamine to a lesser extent.

In terms of dopamine, the quickest way to send dopamine lower for a few days is via a dopamine agonist, as your brain compensates in the first few days by pulling back dopamine production. For me, low dopamine was associated with –

- A lack of pleasure
- A lack of optimism about future events
- An inability to feel excited
- Feeling more irritable than low serotonin did
- Waking up in the middle of the night (However this could have been specific to the pharmaceutical I used)

This experience roughly correlates to what we read in the scientific literature and what we see when patients report their experiences. The main exception was my complete absence of anxiety, which felt rather strange. Whenever I usually get a bit run down or go through a stressful period, I tend to get a little anxious (Stress depletes serotonin). So it felt rather strange to feel a bit low yet experience no anxiety.

However I think it is important to point out that lower dopamine caused by pramipexole is only an issue for the first few days, as with chronic treatment (past say, the first week of start-up) dopaminergic neurotransmission tends to *increase*. Note that I said dopaminergic neurotransmission, not actual dopamine.

Pramipexole (and related dopamine agonists such as cabergoline and ropinirole) mimic the action of dopamine at specific receptors (usually D2, D3 and D4). If you suffer from restless legs or have Parkinson's disease, the first few (often unpleasant) few days should never be a factor in deciding whether to continue or initiate treatment.

This information can be used to allow you to get a greater level of clarity around your mind-state before you see a professional who will be able to offer genuine insight into your predicament. Many people see a therapist without a clear idea of their actual mind state, aside from the general feeling that they are depressed or anxious. Knowing whether dopamine is your problem or whether serotonin is the culprit can be crucial as it dictates the type of treatment you may receive. Giving bupropion to someone with low serotonin or an SSRI to someone with dopamine-related problems can be disastrous, so it can be extremely useful to get a degree of clarity around this point.

Endogenous Opioids

Endorphins, enkephalins and dinorphines

Endorphins (the word stands for *endogenous morphine*) get all the limelight, however there are two more, lesser-known endogenous opioids – enkephalins and dinorphines. Most people vaguely know that "endorphins are your natural pain killers" (which is true), however most people are unaware of the vital and central role these opioids play in your mental wellbeing – not just your pain sensing (*nociceptive*) system.

The story behind their discovery is a fascinating one. For years scientists knew that inside our brains are receptors perfectly designed for activation by opiates like morphine and codeine. However clearly our brains have not evolved specific receptors with the sole purpose of getting us high on morphine! Most of our brains evolved in parts of the world far from any source of opium poppies. This triggered a mad rush to find the endogenous opioids that these receptors were designed to be activated by. Almost simultaneously, two separate groups of scientists discovered endorphins and enkephalins, which, at the time, was viewed as an incredibly important discovery.

Each of the three main endogenous opioids (I will just refer to them as opioids from now on) activate a different sub-type of the opioid receptor. Endorphins activate the mu-opioid receptor, enkephalins activate the delta-opioid receptor and dinorphines activate the kappa-opioid receptor. There are even sub-types of the opioids themselves. For example there is alpha-endorphin, beta-endorphin and so on. However for the purposes of this book I will just refer to the three main opioids in general terms.

The best way to explain what these opioids do is to use the example of a life threatening injury in our distant ancestor past. Imagine you have just been gored by a sabre-tooth tiger or woolly mammoth (I am not paleontologist so these are the only two I could think of – I have no idea whether they were even around the same time as man and have no interest in looking it up!). Not only would it be helpful if you had a natural substance your brain secreted to dull the pain, it would also make sense for this substance to calm you down and reduce stress or suffering. This is, in general, what your opioids are for. It is a little known fact that the most direct route to killing stress is to activate opioid receptors. Due to the general hysteria around opiate drugs and their addiction risk, it is rarely ever mentioned what amazing stress-busters these drugs are. If you are stressed out and anxious, your doctor may prescribe a benzodiazepine like alprazolam (Xanax) or diazepam (Valium), however for many people, a small dose of codeine would be a more direct (and less neurotoxic) way to kill stress.

This is perhaps an explanation why some people become hopelessly addicted to strong opiates like heroin, morphine and oxycodone and why others can take painkillers for as long as they have physical pain and then stop without difficultly. Often the difference is the addict has a stressful (either subtly or overtly) existence which is soothed by opiates. However in other cases the addict doesn't have a need to soothe stress, but an inherent dopaminergic issue which creates addictive behaviors. For these people, it is irrelevant whether it is heroin, cocaine or methamphetamine – they are going to become addicted to something.

Another explanation for the appeal of opiates for some people is the theory that some people have dysfunctional opioid systems which are helped by the additional of an opiate drug. For example, some people may not produce enough natural opioids or their receptors may be dysfunctional.

It is also important to point out that your opioid system is closely connected to your other neurotransmitter systems such as serotonin and dopamine. Activating opioid receptors tends to also boost levels of serotonin and dopamine. The best way to think of it is, when you become injured or experience stress, your brain is like a bartender mixing a cocktail of neurotransmitters to sooth the pain and stress, hopefully enabling you to survive, or in the worst case scenario, ensuring you have a comfortable and stress-free death. Everyone's cocktail will have different proportions of serotonin, dopamine, opioids and noradrenaline. Each of these neurotransmitters work synergistically, causing chain reactions amongst each other. For example, brain imaging and post-mortem studies have shown that high serotonin levels tend to go hand in hand with high levels of endorphins.

However opiate drugs have a much stronger dopaminergic component, to the extent that when someone withdraws from heavy opiate use, often by far the worst withdrawal effects are related to the user no longer having their dopamine levels artificially boosted. The worst of these are usually restless legs and longer term, post-acute withdrawal syndrome (or *PAWS*), which involves a lack of ability to feel pleasure (*anhedonia*) caused by low dopaminergic activity.

The symptoms of low endorphin levels

Compared to serotonin, dopamine and noradrenaline, an endorphin deficiency or dysfunction is actually rather rare, in the absence of opiate use. However I believe there may be a key exception to this. I think that adults who experienced chronic or acute stress as a child may be at increased risk of endorphin system dysfunction later in life. As endorphins are key stress-fighters, there is a chance that someone's endogenous opioid system could become dysfunctional after intense demands are put on it through severe or long-lasting stress.

Probably the single greatest indication of low endorphins or dysfunction is (unsurprisingly) poor tolerance to stress. Someone with poor endorphin responsiveness falls apart at the first sign of emotional stress. This is also seen with long term opiate addict, who find themselves completely unable to deal with any stress if they aren't high on their drug of choice.

Another unsurprisingly symptom of dysfunction would be a low threshold for pain or even hyperalgesia, where you find certain things painful that most people would find to be neutral stimuli (like the example of clothes feeling painful or "scratchy").

In general however, endorphin dysfunction doesn't usually occur in isolation. If you have a problem here, you probably also have an issue with one or more of your monoamines, such as serotonin. Therefore in most cases I think the best option is to address other neurotransmitter imbalances first and endorphins should naturally normalize.

How do I boost my endorphin activity?

Drug-based options

Boosting serotonin makes you love everyone. Boosting dopamine and noradrenaline makes you feel a million dollars.

However boosting endorphins makes you feel like you have gone to heaven, riding on a pain-free cloud.

However there a few problems with boosting opioids (or more accurately *agonizing* opiate receptors) with drugs. Firstly, as with anything that feels good and involves dopamine is going to be addictive for some people. However I should also point out that this is nowhere near as common as most people believe. For example, the only study of its kind found that in patients on long term morphine treatment for pain, only 3% displayed any signs of addiction. Remember, addiction and dependency are two separate things. Anyone on long term opiate therapy will become dependent, which means that if and when the opiates are stopped, the patient will experience withdrawal symptoms. Addiction is an infinitely more complicated beast and typically involves destructive and compulsive usage patterns or dosages which are either much larger than needed for pain management or dosage levels which continually escalate. Personally, I find the idea of doctors withholding pain medication for genuine cases where someone is in considerable chronic pain, over a three in one-hundred chance of addiction, quite ridiculous to be honest. At the opposite end of the scale are doctors who hand out strong opiates like candy, when non-opiate alternatives would be more effective. Hopefully there is a sensible middle ground here.

Secondly, there are some adverse consequences from taking opiates for a long period of time or at high doses, however in comparison to many other drugs (particularly illegal drugs), opiates are relatively benign. An expert in the field once explained it as "There are no health consequences from taking opiates, as long as you are happy being constipated and sterile". Long term opiate users mostly adapt to the problem of constipation through various coping strategies (Hint – it usually involves fiber and water), however there are some hormonal problems associated with opiate use, not the least of which is reduced levels of testosterone. Some opiates also impair immune function, so, whilst this class of drug is relatively benign for the brain and body, it is not without consequence.

In short, opiate drugs should generally be reserved for treating pain or as emergency stress-busters in rare circumstances, not for boosting levels of endogenous opioid activity.

Natural and drug-free options

Now for the good news. For most people, boosting levels of your natural, endogenous opioids is relatively easy.

The most obvious and effective way to do so is via cardiovascular exercise (more on this below). You have probably heard of the runner's high, which is apparently triggered by the release of endorphins in response to the pain of exercise. As a side note, this "high" may not be due only to endorphins. In an experiment, researchers gave test subjects a drug that blocks opioid receptors before they engaged in cardiovascular exercise. Surprisingly, the drug only partially blocked runner's high, suggesting the additional involvement of serotonin, dopamine and noradrenaline in this process.

Another great option is yoga, which has also been shown to trigger the release of endorphins via the painful stretching of your muscles and ligaments. In actual fact anything which is painful will release endorphins. If you want to know exactly what endorphins feel like, remember back to the last time you accidentally stubbed your toe on something. As you may recall, whenever something happens which triggers intense pain, after a second or two your brain will release a flood of endorphins, making you feel almost high for a few seconds longer. However this also points to a problem with focusing on endorphins – they don't really last very long – at least in terms of those brief floods in response to injury. However it is important to maintain the natural hum of various endogenous opioids which is constantly at work in the background. Ask an opiate addict how their body feels if they have gone a long time between doses. Everything hurts. Even the sensation of clothes on their skin can hurt. This gives you an indication on how you would feel with no endorphin activity.

If you would like to support your body's natural production of opioids, you can also support this process nutritionally. However as I have pointed out earlier, ramping up the levels of precursors or substances that support any enzymatic process that creates neurotransmitters and neuro-hormones only helps if this is actually an issue for you. Put another way, mega-dosing on the precursors to endorphins is not going to make you high, as your body will always seek to retain homeostasis.

The amino acid d-phenylalanine is vitally important for endorphin production for two reasons. Firstly, endorphins are comprised of d-phenylalanine and a range of other amino acids and secondly, d-phenylalanine inhibits the degradation process of endorphins, keeping levels higher than they otherwise would have been.

Universal Panaceas

How do I increase levels of serotonin, dopamine, noradrenaline and endorphins at the same time, with one easy fix?

There is one activity which reigns supreme in terms of normalizing and optimizing neurochemistry – cardiovascular exercise. Everything you read about exercise being healthy is true and this is particularly the case with exercise. The human brain loves exercise.

Exercise and its effects on the brain and mood is another topic championed by Benjamin Kramer, who, in his book *Jump Start* said -

Study after study has clearly shown that cardiovascular exercise and/or weight training works just as well as antidepressant medication, but with one key advantage - Those subjects who treat their anxiety and depression with exercise tend to stay well, whereas those who treat their depression with medication have a significantly higher relapse rate.

There are a range of theories as to why exercise is such a powerful booster of neurotransmitters and they all may be at least partially correct. As you have probably surmised, whenever I am trying to work out why the human brain does something, I always find it helpful to think back to our evolutionary past. If we look at exercise, your distant ancestors would have typically used intense cardiovascular exercise for one of two purposes – Either to catch dinner or to escape becoming another creature's dinner. Each of these two activities are central to your survival and therefore, the likelihood that you pass on your genes. In this scenario, each of your neurotransmitters has a vital role to play. Naturally, things are more complicated than this simplification, however for illustrative purposes, you can see the following roles for each of these neurotransmitters –

- **Serotonin** – Reduce anxiety, Increase sense of well-being in the event of mortal injury (note that the way the human brain appears to comfort us as we are about to die doesn't increase the chance of us passing on our genes so in this respect, it remains a mystery in terms of function)
- **Dopamine** – Increase confidence, focus, and energy

- **Noradrenaline** – Increased focus, energy, strength
- **Endorphins** – Reduce stress, sooth pain from injury or fatigue

Your brain loves exercise and it is not simply related to neurochemistry, as exercise triggers a whole host of beneficial processes for your brain. One of the most important is the release of brain-derived neurotrophic factor (BDNF), which, as mentioned earlier, acts as a kind of "fertilizer" for the brain, triggering repair and neuronal growth.

If, for whatever reason, you can't engage in cardiovascular exercise, yoga is a great option. In fact, the gentle pain caused by a deep yoga stretch has been shown to powerfully trigger the release of endorphins. I have left some yoga classes feeling like I was on an opiate drug, due to the huge amount of endorphin activity I had triggered.

Eight

Other neurotransmitters and neuro-
hormones

Whilst the focus of this book is on serotonin, dopamine, noradrenaline and endogenous opioids, there are other important neurotransmitters which are worth highlighting.

Gamma amino butyric acid (GABA)

GABA is your brain's most important inhibitory neurotransmitter. Glutamate puts the foot on the accelerator and GABA is the brake. If you are like most people, at least once or twice you have acutely felt the effects of GABA – benzodiazepine sedatives (or benzos, as they are commonly referred to) like Xanax and Valium work by boosting the activity of GABA, leading to reduced anxiety and eventually, sleep.

This is why this class of drug is the most potent treatment (excluding barbiturates, which I won't get started on...) for anxiety possible. If you boost GABA levels enough, it is virtually impossible to feel anxious.

However GABA is associated with the same problems (and more) as dopamine – Boosting GABA quickly develops tolerance and then leads to addictive behavior. Some people believe benzos to be as addictive as heroin. There is also another major, and more important, downside to boosting GABA with drugs like benzos – They tend to be neurotoxic in higher doses for extended people. If you ever saw someone who has abused benzos for a long period of time you would be shocked. These people are completely fried. This is not a path you want to go down.

Probably the only non-neurotoxic way I know of to boost GABA is via anti-convulsive medications like gabapentin (Neurontin) and pregabalin (Lyrica). In fact, because these drugs can prevent glutamate toxicity (Where glutamate levels are overactive, damaging neurons), there is an argument to suggest that for some people, they are neuroprotective. The key seems to be that these types of drugs don't boost GABA directly. They actually boost GABA by suppressing glutamate. To use the car analogy again, benzos put the foot hard on the brake, whereas drugs like Lyrica slow the car by taking the foot off the accelerator.

In general, like endogenous opioids, I am not really a fan of targeting GABA directly. If you have problems with GABA you almost always have an underlying serotonin issue, as they are very closely interrelated. According to author L. Ciranna in the study *Serotonin as a Modulator of Glutamate- and GABA-Mediated Neurotransmission: Implications in Physiological Functions and in Pathology* (How's that for a mouthful?) in the journal *Current Neuropharmacology*, serotonin *"...exerts a very complex modulatory control over glutamate- and GABA-mediated transmission, involving many subtypes of 5-HT receptors and a large variety of effects."* If you want to fix GABA, you can either start taking a benzo (Not recommended unless you have a severe anxiety disorder) or fix your serotonin signaling through one or more of the various options listed earlier.

Lastly, you may have seen GABA supplements for sale in a health food store. Don't bother. There is very little evidence that oral GABA crosses the blood-brain barrier in any meaningful amounts. GABA is like glutathione in that way – you are better off fixing GABA indirectly.

Glutamate

Now that we have looked at your brain's main "brake", let's move on to the "accelerator".

As glutamate is so abundant and so complicated, I could spend many pages detailing the minutiae of all the various things it does inside your brain. However such an indulgence would be against the spirit of this book which is to keep things to key, interesting points that you can use and apply to your own situation.

There are a range of glutamate receptors, such as the NMDA (*n-methyl d-aspartate*) and AMPA (which stands for, get ready for it, *α-amino-3-hydroxy-5-methyl-4-isoxazolepropionic acid*) receptors. Put simply, your NMDA receptors are involved in a range of functions but are most commonly associated with memory, learning and synaptic plasticity. However this doesn't quite capture the sheer complexity of NMDA receptors. For example, drugs that block (antagonize) NMDA receptors can act as *disassociatives*, such as the street drug PCP (Angel Dust) and the cough suppressant dextromethorphan (Robitussin). This is why some people abuse dextromethorphan by taking large doses (*Robotripping*) or do the same with the horse tranquilizer ketamine. If you block NMDA in sufficiently large doses you will literally lose your grip on reality.

So blocking NMDA receptors must be pretty bad news right? Strangely, no, except perhaps in huge, insane doses. For example, one of the hottest new developments into depression research has been looking at NMDA receptors and their role in depression. There is no prescription drug available which can quickly and effectively treat depression, with one exception. Recently researchers discovered that, if you give ketamine to a depressed person, the depressive symptoms lift almost immediately! This discovery shouldn't be understated as this has been the Holy Grail for some time now. So far this has not translated into a widely available NMDA antagonist antidepressant, however this may change in the near future. Interestingly, in sensible doses, NMDA antagonists actually prevent a type of brain damage known as *glutamatergic excitotoxicity*. In fact, a popular drug for treating Alzheimer's (memantine) helps slow the progression of Alzheimer's, which some researchers believe may be caused by excess glutamate. This is also the reason why the food ingredient monosodium glutamate (MSG) can cause problems for some people (Although this is not as common as most people believe).

AMPA receptors are a little more mysterious but no less important. They are centrally involved in fast synaptic neurotransmission and the process known as long term potentiation (LTP) which underpins learning at the synaptic level. One of the hottest new classes of nootropics, which I covered in my book Brain Hacks, is the AMPAkine class which includes the racetams such as piracetam. Boosting AMPA clearly boosts attention, learning and memory retention.

As you may have guessed, the key to glutamate is dose. A little bit of glutamate is great, a lot of glutamate can be very, very bad. The problem is that there are no really reliable ways to diagnose glutamatergic problems, either high or low. If you are suffering from problems with attention, learning or memory, it can be an option to try a racetam or other AMPAkine and if this fixes things, you have a pretty reliable indicator that your glutamatergic signaling is impaired.

Too much glutamate is even trickier. Clearly you don't want

to wait until you have developed Alzheimer's (It is also implicated in Huntington's, MS and ALS by the way) before you take action. As mentioned earlier, GABA keeps glutamate in check, so if you have had long term problems with low serotonin (and therefore, often low GABA), you could perhaps be a candidate for excess glutamate problems (By the way, just because you have had depression or anxiety, it doesn't mean you have increased risk of developing one of these neurodegenerative illnesses). According to *Psychology Today*, *"having too much glutamate around is to your neurons rather like whipping your horse to go and go and go until you kill it..."* If you think excess glutamate may be an issue, pharmaceuticals are by far the most potent option. In particular, pregabalin (Lyrica), which works by suppressing glutamate and memantine, which is a potent NMDA antagonist, are both effective options. In fact, there is a fascinating study which looked at the neuroprotective effects of combining both of these drugs into a single treatment for fibromyalgia. This study clearly demonstrated that this combination slowed or prevented grey matter loss in the brain associated with excess glutamate.

However fortunately there is one potent and effective way of reducing glutamate toxicity – the almost miraculous substance n-acetylcysteine (NAC). It does everything from heal the liver (it is given to patients in ER who have taken an overdose of acetaminophen/paracetamol, preventing complete liver failure and death), to treating psychiatric illnesses such as OCD and bi-polar disorder (Note – it is typically used as an adjunct treatment in combination with medications, so if you are currently taking medications for these kinds of disorders, don't stop taking them to start NAC. A better option is to discuss with your doctor whether the addition of NAC would be helpful in your case). In terms of glutamate, NAC reduces the release of glutamate through a fairly convoluted series of steps in your brain. Combined with the fact that NAC also boosts levels of glutathione (probably the single most important substance in your body for scavenging free radicals and slowing the aging process), it is potentially one of the most potent brain health supplements available.

Acetylcholine

Acetylcholine, like glutamate, is a key neurotransmitter for controlling aspects of arousal and attention, however in a slightly different way. Acetylcholine is actually distributed all throughout your body and brain, where is controls a range of functions such as muscle control and reward behavior. Acetylcholine is possibly the prototypical neurotransmitter in the classic understanding of a substance that is used to send messages from one part of the brain to another, or to the peripheral nervous system. For example, if you decide to pick up a glass of water, there will be a long chain of acetylcholine signaling where the release of acetylcholine is followed by that acetylcholine binding to their receptors, which triggers more release and so on, down the chain, until it results in a muscular contraction that enable you to pick up that glass of water.

There are two main sub-types of acetylcholine receptors – muscarinic and nicotinic. As you may have guessed, nicotinic receptors are so-called because they are activated by nicotine in tobacco. The activation of the nicotinic receptor by nicotine is not directly related to why people smoke. Activating the nicotinic receptor with nicotine triggers the release of other neurotransmitters including dopamine, which is responsible for the pleasure of smoking. Similarly, muscarinic receptors are named after muscarine, a substance which potently activates them.

It is best to think of acetylcholine as one of the types of electricity your body uses to function. To give you a sense of how important acetylcholine is, many venomous creatures kill prey (and humans) by blocking the animal's acetylcholine system (Anything that blocks this process is known as *anticholinergic*). A lack of cholinergic activity is also associated with Alzheimer's disease, however this link is not proven and attention recently has switched to the Amyloid hypothesis which involves the build-up of plaque in parts of the brain.

As acetylcholine is involved in arousal and muscular activity, anticholinergic drugs tend to be sedating. Many of the older tricyclic antidepressants such as amitriptyline, which tend to knock people out like a light, do so mainly as anticholinergics.

If you experience problems with arousal, attention and other cognitive problems, you could have problems with acetylcholine.

☐

115

Fortunately, you have a range of non-pharmaceutical options available if you want to give acetylcholine a boost. The most potent option is the racetam class of supplements mentioned earlier. As well as boosting glutamate, they also work by giving your acetylcholine a nice bump. My second favorite option is acetyl-l-carnitine (ALCAR), a form of the amino acid l-carnitine which is able to cross the blood-brain barrier and boost acetylcholine.

Substance P

Substance P is another important neurotransmitter that barely gets a mention, however for some people it can be the source of their problems, particularly if those problems include poor tolerance to stress and exaggerated pain response. Substance P is a neuropeptide involved in the transmission of pain, sending messages from around your entire body back to your brain, telling it if you are injured or have something you should be aware of. Being pain free is actually a dangerous thing, like the people with the disorder *congenital insensitivity to pain*, who can't feel pain and consequently end up losing limbs or dying before their time.

Because substance P sends pain messages back to your central nervous system, if things go awry or become dysfunctional you can either feel pain that is not related to an actual injury (such as neuropathic pain) or not feel the pain you should, causing potentially serious injuries to stay outside your awareness. However in general, neuropathic pain is really the main problem that can be caused by substance P, as disorders involving suppressed pain response are incredibly rare in this context.

If you suppress substance P, you dull pain, however suppressing substance P is only weakly effective for treating pain associated with actual, physical problems (such as inflammation or osteoarthritis). Probably the most common substance P related disorder is fibromyalgia, which is associated with widespread pain that is neuropathic in origin. However it is still unclear whether fibromyalgia is caused by or causes increased levels of substance P.

As we saw in the section on endogenous opioids, pain and stress are innately linked and we see a similar situation with substance P. The best way to think of substance P and its relationship to both pain and stress, let's again cue up the wavy music and gaze back into our ancestral past. Chances are, if you were injured, you were also in a stressful situation that required fine-tuned senses and increased arousal to get you out of trouble. Or, to go back the other direction, if you were experiencing severe stress, it is likely that bodily harm was either a risk or imminent, so substance P levels get ramped up to put your senses on full alert. However, transfer this system to modern-day man with severe stress often unrelated to physical harm, it sets us up for chronically elevated substance P levels, leading to pain-related conditions. Substance P is not raised during mild stress. It only really starts peaking when stress levels are severe or chronic.

Understandably, because substance P is part of your danger-sensing apparatus, chronically elevated levels are associated with sleep disorders and possibly anxiety or depression.

If you want to see substance P in action, just rub some hot chili on your skin. Feel that burning sensation even though your skin is not burning? That is the capsaicin in chilies triggering the release of substance P. However this also points to an interesting property of these kinds of "hot" foods like chili and cayenne pepper. If you consume them regularly, in decent doses, you gradually deplete substance P and this can help improve some pain conditions like the various neuralgias. Cayenne pepper is also available as a supplement which can be effective for bringing down substance P levels. Another surprising ingredient for gently bringing down substance P levels is ginger, so if you suffer from neuropathic pain and have problems with digestion, ginger supplements (or reasonable doses of fresh ginger) could be a no-brainer.

In terms of pharmaceuticals, the only commonly available medication that brings down substance P that I know of is our old friend pregabalin (Lyrica – yes this medication does a lot of different things in the body and brain).

Conclusion

Like it or not, much of our conscious experience is dictated by our neurochemistry. Have you ever paused to think how, one minute someone can view their life as worthless or have a poor self-image, only to take a drug such as cocaine or heroin and immediately have a completely different perspective? Or one minute be in mental and physical pain, take an opiate drug (which doesn't do anything to the actual cause of the pain itself, and suddenly you are in heaven. Neurochemicals are powerful little things.

The problem however, is if we focus too much on neurochemicals alone. That spurt of dopamine is your reward (or anticipation of a reward) for something tangible like an achievement of some sorts, focusing on the dopamine alone is like focusing only on the reward and not on the path that will get you to your reward.

I have always found that the best strategy is to put in place whatever you need to in order to normalize any neurochemical issue (medication, lifestyle changes etc.) and then focus on getting on with enjoying a normal life that is in accordance with the principles of neurochemical optimization. Obsessing too much over your neurochemicals is a sure-fire way to unhappiness. Your efforts to boost particular neurotransmitters should be treated like an investment. Spend plenty of time initially working out what your issue is and how to address it, then put it away in the bank and get on with life.

Another problem with obsessing over neurochemistry is that, if you reduce everything to neurochemicals, it can take some of the magic out of life. There is nothing I dislike more than scientists desperately trying to explain near-death experiences in terms of neurochemistry. This actually achieves nothing except test the faith of those trying to be strong when faced with their own mortality. Same goes for love. It drives me crazy when scientists try to explain love as being purely explainable through neurochemistry like oxytocin and serotonin. Love is more than neurochemistry.

So clearly it is a question of balance. Become informed of exactly how your electric brain works so that you know how to live a life which ensures you have the perfect neurochemistry for joy, love, motivation and strength.

Oh, before I forget...

If you enjoyed this book and think others might benefit, please consider leaving a helpful review on www.Amazon.com.

While you are there, please check out my author page, where you can find all of my books, including my best-selling book on slowing the process of cellular aging, *The Methuselah Project - How the science of anti-aging can help you live happier, longer and stronger.*

And finally, Benjamin Kramer has just sent me a copy of the brand-new, completely revised edition of his popular book *Medications for Anxiety & Depression*, which is now a 240 page "encyclopedic" look at every conceivable drug used in mood disorders. Whilst I must admit I have only so far made it half-way, due to time constraints, what I have read is amazingly comprehensive (and I am not just saying that because this book you have just read was name-checked several times – I promise!). Considering that there will be substantial overlap between those reading this book and those interested in Benjamin's book, I thought I should mention it in case you are currently in the process of looking at the need for some form of pharmaceutical assistance.

Made in the USA
Las Vegas, NV
04 April 2024

88207137R00069